stronger

Megan Vickers

stronger

the honest guide to healing and rebuilding after pregnancy and birth

GREEN TREE
LONDON · OXFORD · NEW YORK · NEW DELHI · SYDNEY

GREEN TREE
Bloomsbury Publishing Plc
50 Bedford Square, London, WC1B 3DP, UK
29 Earlsfort Terrace, Dublin 2, Ireland

BLOOMSBURY, GREEN TREE and the Green Tree logo are trademarks of
Bloomsbury Publishing Plc

First published in Great Britain 2021
Copyright © Megan Vickers, 2021

Megan Vickers has asserted her right under the Copyright, Designs and Patents Act, 1988,
to be identified as Author of this work

For legal purposes the Acknowledgements on p. 266
constitute an extension of this copyright page

A catalogue record for this book is available from the British Library

Library of Congress Cataloguing-in-Publication data has been applied for

ISBN: TPB: 978-1-4729-8630-6; eBook: 978-1-4729-8629-0

2 4 6 8 10 9 7 5 3 1

Typeset in Minion Pro by Deanta Global Publishing Services, Chennai, India
Printed and bound in Great Britain by CPI Group (UK) Ltd, Croydon CR0 4YY

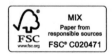

MIX
Paper from
responsible sources
FSC
www.fsc.org
FSC® C020471

To find out more about our authors and books visit www.bloomsbury.com
and sign up for our newsletters

Contents

Introduction

Maybe you've picked up this book because you're finally done with wetting yourself laughing and it's no longer funny. Perhaps your already-mum friends brought it along to your baby shower to give you an eye-opening account of what recovery from birth is really like and you thought it was a joke. Or possibly it's gone past the point where you can ask your midwife to explain exactly what she means when she talks about your pelvic floor and 'Kegel' exercises. This guide will 'bare all' and reveal all the questions you didn't know you had, as well as answering those you were too embarrassed to ask.

Whether you're preparing for motherhood, have recently become a mother or are weeks, months or many years down the line, it is never too late to heal and rebuild. Growing and birthing a baby is a magical but brutal process. Things we took for granted change drastically over this time, from how our hormones communicate and control us, to the way we breathe and move, to how often we pee and poo. We sometimes forget to acknowledge these vast changes or forgive ourselves when our bodies stubbornly refuse to spring back into pre-pregnancy shape. We can call this the fourth trimester, the post-natal period or getting our body back, but if we don't use this time to consciously heal and rebuild our bodies then we may stay in this phase for years, if not a lifetime.

After pregnancy, the truth is that problems with our body, and particularly our pelvic floors, will affect most of us. Pelvic floor weakness is a taboo topic and this part of our body is not treated with the care it deserves. You might share a laugh with another mum about having to cross your legs when you sneeze or nip behind a bush to pee mid-run, but behind closed doors you're probably devastated by this. Most of us would rather die than openly discuss fanny farting, poo stains in our underwear or not making it to the bathroom in time. We would sooner cover up and change our whole wardrobe before talking to our doctor about still looking pregnant months later, anxiety or unhappiness around our changed shape, and negative feelings towards our baby as a result.

To be honest, though, how many of us really understand what pelvic floor exercises are, and know how they help and how to perform them properly? How many of us could competently navigate our nether regions even before the changes that come with pregnancy and birth? I'm going to teach you about your body and how it functions in order to make it strong, and help you optimise your overall health and fitness. I get it. I'm the physio, so why do you need to learn how your body works? Can't I just tell you what to do? Think of healing and rebuilding your body as if you were completing a jigsaw puzzle. There are many ways of doing it – the edges first, outwards from the corners or matching colours – but whatever way you do it, isn't it easier to know what the final picture should look like? What is it that you're trying to piece together? You're not expected to memorise this either. Look back at these lessons in anatomy at any time, just like coming across a tricky piece of puzzle and looking at the picture on the box to work out where it should go.

So what does healing and rebuilding actually mean?

Even relatively straightforward pregnancies and births can stretch our bodies to their limits, and often beyond. After carrying and delivering children, it is vital that we allow time for our bodies to repair and our hormones to return to normal-ish levels. In order to restrengthen our pelvic floors, tummies, pelvises and spines, we must *protect, stabilise and rehabilitate* each part. This is my post-natal mantra and you will see these words frequently here, because these steps are the secret to rebuilding after any injury.

It begins with *protect*. To protect is to keep from harm and after the birth of our babies our bodies are vulnerable, but – until now – there was not enough clarity on how to care for ourselves and avoid post-birth injuries. And it's not just immediately after the birth of our babies that we need to protect our bodies, but also before our babies are born and for many moons after. In the excitement of a new baby a mother's recovery is often overlooked, but your care, support and protection are just as important as your baby's.

Needing to duck out of gym classes to wee, a feeling of heaviness in your vagina after running to work and an acceptance of painful constipation are all warning signs and examples of experiences that we need to prevent and recover from rather than adapt to and compensate for.

Alongside protect we need to *stabilise*. To rebuild and restore we first need a stable base to work from. Just like building a strong house, if we don't set

8

it on solid, stable foundations it won't stay strong for long. Some mothers I work with have done much to rebuild and strengthen their bodies, but have left out protection and stabilisation, meaning that their foundations remain weaker. Only once we have addressed those issues can we truly *rehabilitate* and restore our strength.

Protect, stabilise and rehabilitate are the tools you'll need for this journey, so let's get started.

Protect: Uncross your legs! I'm guilty of this all the time, even though I know it twists my pelvis, and makes my pelvic floor wonky and my back crooked, so even I need to set myself reminders. Start with both of your feet on the floor, raise your bottom a little higher than your knees by sitting on a cushion and check your back is fully supported, so that you can relax and don't need to cross your legs to get comfy.

Stabilise: Find your best posture. This is more than just propping yourself in the best position, it comes down to switching on your muscles. Try to grow as tall as you can, as though your head is a helium balloon floating up to the ceiling. Now imagine you're wearing your favourite necklace and show if off proudly, letting your breastbone lift up and out of your chest. Notice how you're no longer slouched, slumped or dependent on your chair to hold you up. This posture comes from your own stability and strength.

Rehabilitate: Now you're ready to exercise your pelvic floor, which is a group of muscles slung like a hammock, stretching from the bone at the front of your pelvis to your tail at the back, and across from side to side. Its job is to support our bladder, bowel and womb, and help us wee, poo and have sex when we want to, as well as creating the birth canal. However, perhaps its most important job is to give us core strength. It literally pulls our pelvis together and provides our whole body with support from the ground up. Had no idea, huh? I think very few of us actually know what or where our pelvic floor is, or how to work it properly. Fear not, that's all about to change...

To find and feel it, think of your muscular pelvic floor as an elevator. Most of us can pinch our pelvic floor closed to stop wee or wind escaping. This is the equivalent of the elevator doors closing. You are using the muscles on the outside and may feel, and even see, the openings for your pee and poo pipes close. However, just like your elevator, it hasn't gone anywhere yet. You've shut the doors, but there is a whole lot more that this muscle needs to be able to do, so hold the elevator doors tightly shut and try to pull the openings for your pee and poo pipes up and inside you, as though that elevator is moving high up into your pelvis. Take your elevator up to the first floor and hold it there. Now, without clenching your bottom or pulling your tummy in, take your pelvic floor elevator to the penthouse. Pause at the top... then slowly lower your elevator down, releasing your muscles. Finally release the pinch, open the doors of your elevator and relax your pelvic floor fully. Well done! That's the first task ticked off. Don't worry if you couldn't feel it or found this impossible. There are plenty more tasks in the coming chapters, but until we get to those practise this every day and you will be surprised how much better you get at lifting your elevator and maybe even reaching your penthouse.

The drawbacks of pregnancy and birth that we're going to tackle, improve and resolve are:

- **Changes in your posture:**How we sit and stand affects our whole system. Your posture changes the position of your bladder and womb on top of the pelvic floor, and the position and functioning of the pelvic floor itself. Muscle length and strength is something that we can address to change posture, as well as spinal mobility. To accommodate growing a baby, our pelvis and rib cage naturally widen in pregnancy and birth. They may or may not 'close' on their own, no matter how many months or years after giving birth you are. This can mean pain and other problems now or years down the line. It's essential that we strengthen to deal with these changes (see task 2 on page 39 for more on this).

- **Pelvic floor tightness or weakness**: This includes not only leaking wee or poo (incontinence), but also being desperate to go (urgency), pain, oversensitivity or diminished sensation altogether. As it's made up of many muscles and goes through many changes in pregnancy and birth, it's normal for some parts of the pelvic floor to work harder than others. In order to have a 'strong' pelvic floor we need all the muscles to work together, to have the capacity to both contract and relax fully. Many problems women encounter after birth, such as wetting our knickers, are blamed on pelvic floor weakness, but in fact stem from pelvic floor *tightness.* A pelvic floor that is too tense will struggle to work harder when it needs to and will struggle to relax fully. We need this to pee, poo and have pleasurable sex. Tense (high tone or hypertonic) pelvic floors are more common than you might think and I'll help you strengthen *and* relax yours (tasks 3 on page 55 and 4 on page 58 will do this).

- **Painful birth injuries**: Cuts or tears to our perineum (the part between our vagina and anus) or Caesarean scars are intimately connected to emotional trauma from difficult birth experiences. The connection between our physical and emotional selves is deep, but too often we are left to heal on our own. If we don't heal as we expect then the emotional wounds can affect many aspects of our lives. Often scars heal following infection or re-opening and can heal tightly. This can make them painful to touch or impact how we sit, go to the loo or have penetrative sex. These physical side-effects can be painful reminders of birth that hinder our complete recovery. This doesn't need to be the case. Here you'll find all you need to know about recovery from Caesarean and perineal trauma after birth (tasks 6, 7 and 8 on pages 83–97 focus on this).

- **Pelvic organ prolapse**: This is when the vaginal walls are weakened, thinned or stretched and the back passage, womb or bladder press down into the vaginal space. It is truly awful to be told that your vagina is caving in on itself at any age, but no more so when you are a new mum and want to feel your strongest. Knowing what will help and what will worsen this injury is a total minefield. It can feel impossible to know what's right, especially when you have a new baby to care for. With my protect, stabilise and rehabilitate mantra I'll lead you by the hand through this journey and it's one which I have taken myself to feel stronger (task 9 on page 118 deals with pelvic organ prolapse).

- **Problematic tummies**: Pregnancy inevitably stretches our tummy muscles as they make room for our expanding uterus and growing baby. This will weaken and may even separate our abdominal muscles. Their strength, appearance and ability to be our 'core support' is compromised as a result. After birth these muscles naturally shorten again, but don't always automatically return to their pre-pregnancy shape. Abdominal, or core strength is essential for posture, spinal support and almost every movement we take. The exercises and advice in this book will help you to get them back to full strength (go to tasks 12, 13, 14 and 15 that can be found on pages 157–173).

- **Back and pelvic pain**: In pregnancy this is often called PGP (pelvic girdle pain), which is pain in your back or bottom, or SPD (symphysis pubis dysfunction), which is pain in the bone under your pubic hair. As our bodies change so enormously to accommodate new life, it's no surprise that this comes with painful adaptations to our muscles and joints that do not always resolve once our babies are born. We should not assume that our bodies can spring back to their pre-pregnancy position and shape all of their own accord. Most will need a little coaxing, some postural stretches and a big serving of strength-based training (this is covered in tasks 10 and 11 on pages 140–43).

- **Understanding how to safely return to exercise and sex**: Maybe you feel OK right now, but are anxious about a new pregnancy, returning to exercise or doing too much too soon. But what is too much too soon? Our births and our recoveries are unique, as are our lifestyles and dreams, but preparation and knowledge is key to achieving what we desire. There may be new ideas here that you've never considered, so why not embrace the challenge and see if you can achieve your goals? (Tasks 18 and 19 on pages 211–223 will help you do this.)

What about my six-week check?

This list was covered by your GP at your six-week check, right? They examined you inside and out, and covered all these issues? You weren't in a rush, stressed by a crying baby or too embarrassed to share everything you felt? I'm going to guess no…

For many of us the six-week check is a long-anticipated appointment at which we hope to be told we are back to normal and can be signed off, even if we know we don't *feel* quite the same. However, if it's not performed thoroughly and doesn't include all of the points above then this well-timed and well-meant check-up can feel like the end of the recovery road; that this is as good as we can expect to feel. But the truth is our bodies still have much healing and rebuilding to do. Our GPs are general practitioners, not experts in pregnancy, birth and all the changes that these bring. It's like going to the supermarket for a bespoke birthday cake or a corner shop for a craft beer – you might find what you're looking for, but more often than not you will need to go elsewhere. Instead of considering the six-week check as a *sign off*, we must use this opportunity to connect to the help that we need. You need to take the first step by making the initial call or showing up, but, rather like the operator at one of those old-fashioned telephone exchanges, your GP knows what services are available and how to plug you in to that help. And just like that telephone operator, your GP is always available. You can ask for their help not just at six weeks, but at any time. You don't deserve to suffer in silence and it's your right to say, 'No. I am still in pain. This doesn't feel right. I'm not happy.'

When to ask for help:

- You are leaking urine, wind or poo after the acute inflammation of birth has settled. Anything longer than 2–3 weeks is not normal.
- You are unable to pee or poo properly after the same time period.
- You feel as if there's a tampon coming out when you're not wearing one or you can see or feel something – often described as an egg – at the opening of your vagina. This is what a prolapse feels like.
- You experience pain in your tummy, pelvis, back, bladder, vagina (what's on the inside), vulva or perineum (what you can see on the outside) that doesn't resolve within the same 2 –3 weeks.
- You feel pain or loss of sensation during sex once your scars have healed. This normally takes a maximum of six weeks.
- You feel numbness or pain around your Caesarean scar after healing has occurred. It can take 12 weeks to return to normal.
- You feel low in mood, sad, anxious, depressed or low in energy, regardless of how much rest you have.

What to ask for:

- A referral for women's health physiotherapy, which is available on the NHS in most areas of the UK, and in most medical centres worldwide.
- An appointment with a gynaecologist if you think – or are told –you have a prolapse, so that you can discuss the extent of your injury and rehabilitation options.

- Oestrogen cream if you are breast feeding (or menopausal) to help with your pelvic floor muscle tone.
- Laxatives or stool (poo) softener to ensure that you can poo daily, without pain or straining.
- Mental health support and blood tests if you feel lower in energy or mood than what you feel is normal for you. Your iron, thyroid and vitamins D and B will need to be tested, as well as your blood sugar, which, when low, can also be responsible for changes in our mood.

Women frequently reach out to me for help after they've tried to talk to their midwife, health visitor or GP and haven't been satisfied with the answers. I was motivated in part to write this book to call out the untruths and address the flippancy with which women's health is often regarded in the medical world. For example, women I know have been told:

- You have a prolapse – don't do any exercise, ever.
- You've just had a baby – you should be lying down with your legs in the air and doing nothing (my GP said this to me three weeks after my first baby was born!).
- Everybody leaks – just wear a pad.
- You had your baby six weeks ago and you are no longer post-partum, so you can return to everything you were doing before (the same GP said this at my six-week check).
- You may have pelvic discomfort all day long and can't open your bowels, but your prolapse isn't *that* bad.
- You should do pelvic floor exercises all the time – while you're feeding your baby, waiting at traffic lights, watching TV… Spoiler alert: you shouldn't. This is like saying that if you want a flatter tummy you should just pull it in. Strength training is a focused and progressive regime, as we'll see over the coming chapters.

If you've been told something similar, you probably knew the advice didn't feel right for you, but had no idea where to go next. In an ideal world these issues would be covered during your ante-natal journey, in your birth preparation classes, midwifery appointments or at your six-week post-natal check, rather than leaving you to ask Google.

However well-intentioned they are, those 'bladder weakness' incontinence pad adverts send us the message that these conditions don't warrant treatment. It is as though wetting ourselves is normal and part and parcel of a woman's existence, and we simply have to accept it. The ads fail to acknowledge the embarrassment and social stigma of reporting incontinence and the associated depression. They forgive the medical system for under-recognising and under-treating these conditions. The pads should come with a caveat that they are to be used alongside medical treatment and physiotherapy rehabilitation, as a stopgap between injury and recovery.

It's time we refused to keep quiet about our pain and problems after pregnancy and birth. Injuries to any other part of our body would be investigated and cared for, and we should expect nothing less for injuries sustained in the process of motherhood. If we consider every birth, vaginal tear or Caesarean scar as we do a sports injury, the need to heal and rebuild would be obvious. Not only this, but diagnosis would be easy, with scans and X-rays at our disposal via emergency departments. Injuries sustained in birth often go undiagnosed, aren't investigated and remain unhealed. But until healthcare for mothers is successfully prioritised, let's cradle our own broken parts together and use this book to grow even stronger than we were before.

So how common are problems after pregnancy and birth and can we really fix them?

In short, very common and, yes, we can. Symptoms of a problematic pelvic floor can be mild or devastatingly severe. These include leaking wee, wind or poo; not being able to empty your bladder or constantly need to go; urgency; constipation; wetting the bed; involuntary queefing (fanny farts); pelvic pain; pelvic organ prolapse; lack of orgasms and pain with sex. That might read like a terrifying list, but I want you to know that you do not need to put up with these issues, there is A LOT we can do to change these things – pelvic floor strengthening is low risk and the most effective way of resolving these issues – and you are not alone. Here are the stats:

- 50% of pregnant women will experience lower back pain in pregnancy and, without treatment, 25% of those will still be suffering from pain one year after delivery.
- 100% of women at full-term pregnancy will have some degree of tummy muscle overstretch and 30% will have a separation known as diastasis recti abdominis muscle (DRAM – see page 154).
- 90% of first-time vaginal births will result in some degree of vaginal or perineal tear and sometimes an episiotomy (a cut through the pelvic floor muscles to make the birth easier).
- More than 25% of UK births are abdominal (via Caesarean section), which is major surgery.
- 30-50% of mums will wet themselves a little – or a lot.
- 3-7% of post-natal women will not be in full control of their bowels and will leak poo, while 25% will have no control over their wind (farting). This is no wonder when it's the anal sphincter nerves which undergo the most strain in the second stage of labour.
- 50% of mothers will have some degree of pelvic organ prolapse by the time they reach menopause. This needn't be as scary as it sounds, because knowing the correct pelvic floor exercises and how to do them properly means you can improve and in many cases resolve your symptoms.

While more than a third of women suffer with urinary incontinence, only half of these will seek advice and treatment from medical professionals. I am a firm believer that treatment and exercise should be our go-to approach, not incontinence pads. We must spread the message that these issues can be fixed and it's time to treat what we pretend not to see.

It's good to work directly with a physiotherapist, but accessing help is a big problem and women's health physiotherapy can be hard to come by in the UK. In much of Europe a course of physiotherapy after having a baby is standard practice for all. In France, for instance, you are discharged home with your baby and a prescription for a course of six physical therapy appointments to rebuild your strength. However, in the UK access to the right professional help to support your body can be a postcode lottery, so I'm sharing everything with you that I've learned through my own research, listening to and treating the hundreds of women I've had the pleasure of working with, and my own personal experiences. All you need to know and do is here, explained step by step.

About me

My professional title is Pelvic Obstetric and Gynaecological Physiotherapist, but my friends call me the Fanny Physio. My colleagues and I assess and treat any pain and problems in the pelvic region, which includes everything inside a pair of your biggest knickers, from your genitalia on the outside down to your deepest pelvic floor muscles, bladder, bowel and even your spine. We are the first port of call when things feel or work differently 'down there', and our knowledge and tools are essential to every woman for the prevention, as well as the treatment, of injury, birth-related or not. The women I treat often tell me that exercise before babies was all about their looks, whereas their motivation for training after pregnancy and birth is based on how they feel and the benefits that their physical strength has on their entire wellbeing.

I set up my own rehab space, Four Sides London, in 2017 with my husband, James, and my business partners, Claire and Paul. I treat men and women, and am passionate about rehabilitating the whole body. I have dedicated much of my working life to pelvic pain, pregnancy and post-natal exercise, and am a crusader for understanding and rehabilitating our pelvic floors. My own body, pregnancies and post-natal journeys have also been incredibly valuable learning tools. I wrote this book in order to pass on all that I have learnt as both a physiotherapist and a mother.

I have grown and given birth to two girls and they have been by my side in every step of this ongoing journey. I have enjoyed one pain-free pregnancy and endured one difficult pregnancy, rife with pelvic girdle pain. I have had both an 'unnatural' birth (medical induction, episiotomy and ventouse) and a natural delivery. My first post-natal journey was a shock – I never thought that I of all people would sustain a birth injury! Despite this being my occupation, I felt totally unprepared for my own post-natal rehabilitation. My second post-natal journey, on the other hand, was highly regimented. I did everything by the book – now this book! – and I felt in control of my healing body. I knew when to push myself not based on the passing of time, but by what I could achieve. I have also rehabilitated myself after abdominal surgery (a hernia) and know the pain and limitations of a raw tummy wound.

I have had post-natal depression twice, and know that how our bodies feel has a huge impact on our emotional wellbeing, because not only have I witnessed it but I have been through it myself. It is OK to not be OK, and it is more than OK to be working on it. This is an ongoing journey for both body and mind. I am still learning and value the experience of every client and the challenges these bring. I am privileged to share the secrets and tools of my trade; to reveal to everyone the power of women's health physiotherapy and the building blocks to healing after pregnancy and birth that should be accessible to all.

It's never too late to rebuild that strength and confidence in our physical ability, and to change the statistics I quoted above – I certainly hope that when my girls are grown up, that things will be significantly different. I want to enable you to feel strong and capable; empowered to invest in your physical wellbeing; and able to self-care, heal and rebuild your strength completely. This is the same advice I pass on to my clients on a daily basis and it's the same programme that I have used myself. I am often asked, 'Why didn't anyone ever tell me this before?' Settle in. This is for you.

1. Our bodies: My favourite parts

Understanding our body and the changes it may have gone through in pregnancy and birth is fundamental to being in control of our own healing and rebuilding. These next few pages will help you appreciate and connect with it, so you can take care of yourself for the rest of your life. My goal is for you to become an expert in your body and all its quirks, but before we can address how to fix it, we need to know what's there. Bear with me and I promise it will be worth it!

Our bodies are complicated and amazing, and while this chapter may feel like an anatomy lesson (it kind of is), you could think of it more as a tour of your own home. When we're thinking about the pelvic floor we also need to take into account the bony pelvis that houses it, the muscular walls which surround it and both its energy source and 'control panel'. Think of your pelvis as the foundations, and your spine and rib cage as the framework that the walls are built around. Your pelvic floor muscles make up the ground floor and then your abdominal muscles at the front, which wrap around the sides to meet your spinal muscles at the back, are the walls. Your diaphragm, a muscle which moves in sync with your pelvic floor, intimately linking pelvic floor function to your every breath, is the roof. Finally, there are your nerves and hormones. These are the electrics and your power supply, and they make everything function... or not.

Diane Lee, a physiotherapist and a role model of mine, has a similar analogy for our pelvic floor. She describes the pelvis as our door frame and the muscular pelvic floor as our door. We can spend a lot of time strengthening the 'door', doing our pelvic floor exercises or Kegels, and utilising a whole array of pelvic floor strengthening apparatus (more on Kegels, gadgets and gizmos in chapter 3), but if the door frame is twisted or creaking then the door will never close. As a result, we will struggle to achieve optimal pelvic floor closure or 'lift', leaving us susceptible to pelvic organ prolapse, bladder and bowel mishaps, and pelvic pain. I find this a really useful way to think about the relationship between our bones and our muscles, because it highlights that we need to address the door frame *and* the floor together. To rebuild after pregnancy and birth we need to do some detective work to figure out which parts of our house we need to address to make the whole thing stronger.

The bony pelvis

The three bones of the pelvis form the centre of our bodies. Our pelvic ring connects our upper and lower halves. The pelvis is the base of our spine and forms the foundations for the pelvic floor. This bony structure is frankly

The Bony Skeleton

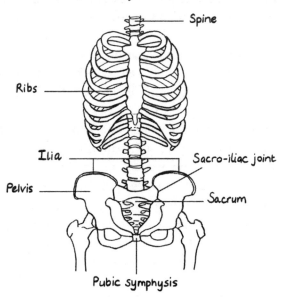

The Ligaments of the Pelvis

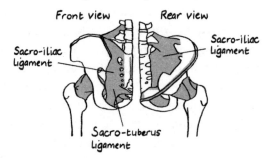

amazing. It is mobile and accommodating, most of our body's movements pass through here and it has kept your baby safe.

The pelvis is made up of three bones and these fit nicely together like a jigsaw puzzle making a perfect ring. Your two pelvic bones are called ilia. You can find their crested tops if you put your hands on your hips. From here your fingers can find the bony nobbles which mark the front of these pelvis bones. Now track your fingers down and together to meet at your pubic area. It is here, at your pubic bone where the two ilia join. Between the two bones sits softer cartilage and this is called the pubic symphysis. When there is pain in this area it can spread outwards and even downwards to the vagina, causing SPD or symphysis pubis dysfunction, which you may have endured during pregnancy. The cartilage is here for shock absorbency and to allow the movement which one continuous bone would not accommodate. The most obvious movement at this joint is when it opens for childbirth, but there are also tiny movements forwards and backwards when we step, walk, run or cross our legs. The gap at the pubic symphysis is normally 3-4mm, but can more than double in pregnancy and birth to up to 9mm. The bigger the steps we take or the larger our baby, then the more movement there is at the pubic symphysis. In pregnancy, if this joint widens too rapidly as a result of hormones, is stretched forcefully as a result of trauma or previous tricky births, or just strained repetitively through movement, then inflammation and pain can creep in. This is when the tiny movements we are normally unaware of when we step, put on our socks or climb stairs can become painful as our muscles struggle to function under these new conditions. There is more on resolving this type of pelvic pain in chapter 7.

Now hands back on your hips with your thumbs pointing backwards. Work them in towards the spine to find the back of the ilia. This is where the pelvis meets the base of the spine, the sacrum, which is the third bone of the pelvis. The joints between each of the ilia and the sacrum are called the sacro-iliac joints. You have one on the left and one on the right. There are corresponding grooves on the sacrum and ilia allowing the sacrum to fit snugly between the two bones, just like a jigsaw piece. The ligaments and muscles which cross the bones work to keep these joints stable as we move.

Stretchy ligaments

Ligaments are tough bands of connective tissue which connect bone to bone. If you've ever looked at one of those life-like skeletons often found in physio and doctor's rooms you may have noticed that the bones are pinned together with wires and screws. Without them the skeleton would be a heap of bones on the floor. The wires and screws create the connection from one bone to the next, keeping the bones in their perfect anatomical position, and in our bodies this is exactly what our ligaments do. The point where the bones join is called a joint and the ligaments provide joint stability. In pregnancy the joints at the back of the pelvis also widen naturally and the sacrum slips down between the ilia to make more space for our growing baby or babies. In childbirth these joints can widen even further and displace the sacrum from its normal locked position. The hormone relaxin makes our ligaments stretch more than normal to enable this to happen.

If you experience pain in the pelvis or lower back it's probably not in the bones themselves, but is more likely to be coming from these soft tissue support structures which are not very accommodating or happy when they're overstretched or overloaded. These structural ligaments can become painful when you're carrying too much weight (yes, a full-term baby counts) or if your movements are repetitive or lopsided. Think about jutting out your left hip to hold a wriggling toddler and keep your right arm free – you lift your left pelvis up to form a convenient resting place for the child and your opposite shoulder moves higher. This stretches and creates tension in the ligaments on the left, and compresses and pinches those on the right.

The most important ligaments to get to know are your sacro-iliac (SI) and your sacro-tuberus (ST). Place your fingers at the top of your bottom and trace this line upwards to the hard bone in the midline of your sacrum. Now move both hands outwards 5cm and you'll feel it becomes less bony, a little gristly and often tender to press. This is the SI ligament and you can track it up either side of your sacrum to the dimples of your lower back. The SI ligament crosses the sacro-iliac joints and not only holds our pelvis together, but is also stretchy enough to allow those little movements that occur with every step we take. The ST ligament connects your spine to the bottom of your pelvis (the ischial tuberosities or sitting bones). You can find this ligament by reaching around with both hands to where your bottom meets your thighs. Press in firmly – you may need to rock backwards and forwards – to find your sitting bones. Now you can track the ST ligament as it runs upwards and inwards to your tailbone (coccyx) at the bottom of your sacrum. You may need to bend forwards or try this in a seated position where this ligament is stretched. It feels like a taut banjo string and may be tender to touch. If the areas you have just mapped out are painful for you, then that's good, because working out what is sore is the first step in fixing it. To ease discomfort in these areas, pay particular attention to the postural and release exercises in task 2 (see page 39).

Our core muscles

So that's ligaments. Next let's find our muscles. The key core muscles are those which make up our abdominal cylinder: its base (the pelvic floor muscles and inner thigh), the front (the abdominals), the back (the spinal and buttock muscles) and the top (the diaphragm.) Together they form a critical hub for stability, control and the development of our breath, bladder, bowel and all our body's movements.

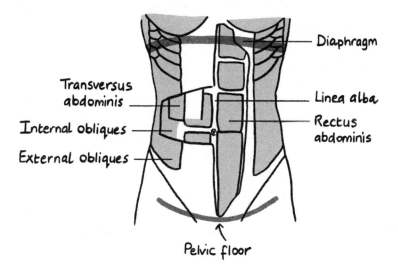

Diaphragm

Transversus abdominis

Linea alba

Internal obliques

Rectus abdominis

External obliques

Pelvic floor

The floor

Let's start at the bottom. The pelvic floor is several layers of muscles slung like a hammock across the floor of the pelvis. Together this group of muscles is called the levator ani (Latin for elevate your anus!). It attaches to the C-shaped ilia bones at the sides, the sacrum and tailbone at the back, and the pubic symphysis at the front, and they even have connections to our thigh bones. If we move or twist these bones the pelvic floor moves and twists too. Like all muscles in the body, when we contract or squeeze the pelvic floor muscles they shorten, our muscle fibres cross over one another and the muscles become dense and taut. This pulls the bones of the pelvic ring – the sacrum at the centre and 2 ilia either side – together and at the same time the pelvic organs – the vagina, uterus, cervix, bladder and bowel – are lifted higher into the pelvis.

There are three key layers of the pelvic floor, each with its own role. The muscles closest to the outside of our bodies are muscular sphincters or circular muscles which pinch our passages closed to control what goes in and out. Where our urine exits there is a urethral sphincter, at our back passage there is an internal anal sphincter which we cannot consciously control (involuntary) and an external anal sphincter which we can clench on demand (voluntary). In my experience most of us can find and tighten these muscles when we're performing pelvic floor exercises, but struggle with the deeper layers of muscles. If we rely on this superficial layer alone then we are only reaching one third of our pelvic floor muscle potential.

The deeper pelvic floor muscles work from our tailbone at the back to our pubic bone at the front, closing down the passages of our bladder, bowel and vagina, lifting our rectum and womb, and pressing the urethra (pee pipe) firmly against the pubic symphysis to stem the flow of urine. Their job is to pull the pelvic hammock taut and lift our pelvic organs high up, away from the openings of our vagina, bowel and bladder, known as our pelvic outlets.

To some degree our pelvic floor muscles are subconsciously tense most of the time. They relax when we need them to, so that we can go to the bathroom, but we don't normally have to think about holding in our wee all day long. Thankfully, our body does this for us… unless, of course, there has been an injury (which can occur during pregnancy and birth). During forceful activities such as sneezing, jumping or running we need greater pelvic floor strength to resist the downward forces which these activities bring. The great news is that, like any muscles in the body, we can train the pelvic floor muscles to become stronger, lift greater loads, respond faster and have better endurance.

The roof

The top of our core cylinder is the diaphragm – a large muscular sheet attached to the inside of our ribcage, breast bone and spine which reflects the pelvic floor muscle below. It's a muscular sheet that contracts and pulls down to draw air into our lungs, and then relaxes and recoils upwards to push air out. The pelvic floor moves in sync with the diaphragm and you may even be able to feel this (don't worry if you can't!). I can still recall the heaviness I felt in my pelvic floor with every in-breath after the birth of my first baby. It made me acutely aware of the injuries I had sustained and that I needed to rebuild.

During pregnancy the ribcage can be stretched outwards by 4cm or more – you probably noticed this in the snug fit of your bra. This adaptation is essential to make space for your growing baby. As the diaphragm and abdominal wall connect to these lower ribs, those 4cm can make a real difference to how these muscles function, not just in pregnancy but afterwards too. Taking a full breath in can become a challenge for the diaphragm and this increased rib circumference also makes it more difficult to close the tummy and pelvic ring after pregnancy. The ribcage is an anchor for the abdominal muscles and so the greater the increase in ribcage circumference during pregnancy, the wider and more significant the tummy muscle separation is. And just like the pelvic floor and pelvis, if we only train the muscles without focusing on the position of the bones, then we are only addressing half of the problem. Tackling the rib cage circumference comes down to good posture, and mid-back and rib mobility, as well as core cylinder strength (there's more to come on this in task 2 on page 39).

My clients are often worried about how to synchronise their breathing in their exercise programmes. I tell them not worry about this yet as it will come later. That's not because it's not important, but that in order to incorporate our breath we need a pelvic floor and abdominal wall that are working in sync and can resist the increase in pressure that comes with changing lung volumes. This is hard if you have a perineal wound from an episiotomy, an abdominal wound from a Caesarean, tummy muscle separation or pelvic organ prolapse. It's far too much to ask our body to relearn core movements at this deep level *and* co-ordinate breathing simultaneously. Master one and the other becomes so much easier. We can't incorporate breath automatically in this relearning process, but should do it separately, honouring the changes that have occurred in our bodies. This is why breath has a chapter all of its own (see chapter 9).

The walls
These run from top to bottom (literally) and across our entire abdomen and include both our abdominals (our abs) at the front and our spinal muscles at

the back. Just like the pelvic floor, the walls have many layers of muscle and connecting tissue stacked on top of one another, each with their own role. The deepest layer is the transversus abdominis, which wraps around the tummy and has connections to the spine and its muscles at the back, to the ribcage and diaphragm at the top, and the pelvic floor and pelvis at the bottom. It may not give as much visible strength as the brickwork on the outside, but think of it as the plasterboard and wallpaper on the inside of your walls – it makes your house a home.

It also looks and acts like a corset. Imagine wearing one of those through pregnancy, after birth and every day thereafter. You probably feel like you'd stand a little taller, breathe a little deeper and move with more control. I'm imagining it now and can't help but 'lift up and in'. During pregnancy this muscle has to stretch not only around your growing uterus and across your baby bump, but also from above, behind and down below as our ribcage, diaphragm, pelvis and pelvic floor all expand. So naturally, because of this stretch, its automatic action is reduced as it becomes less like a tight corset and more like a loose belt. You might think that training this muscle during pregnancy is counterintuitive and restrictive for your growing baby, but this is far from the case.

Training your transversus abdominis throughout pregnancy helps to maintain strength as it stretches, rather than restricting your tummy's expansion altogether. The muscles remain strong to support your baby bump, your posture, breathing, back and pelvic floor. Don't worry if you're reading this after having a baby and have never heard of the transversus abdominis before. If you've never trained it, just imagine that feeling of wearing a muscular corset all day long and what that would do for your movement and posture. It's never too late to wake it up! You can find it, strengthen it and get right back on track at any stage. It's just like starting something new, it takes a little while, but you will become better at it soon enough (you'll learn how shortly in task 1).

Front door

The long muscle stretching down the front of our tummy and over our baby bump as it grows is the rectus abdominis, our 'six pack'. It's true that we all have one and, whether it's visible and rippling on the surface or more hidden, its actions are the same. The rectus abdominis runs as two vertical muscles from the front of your ribcage all the way down to your pubic bone and pubic symphysis. These two muscles are joined in the middle by stiff connective tissue called the linea alba. Both the rectus abdominis muscle and the linea alba stretch as our babies grow in pregnancy. While muscle fibres are built to lengthen and shorten again, connective tissue is not so elastic and the linea alba becomes thin, allowing the two parts of the rectus abdominis to move apart and our baby bump to grow. Almost all women who carry to full term will experience this muscle separation to some degree and for most of us it will start to close from day one after birth. However, for about a third of us, the linea alba becomes too thin and little micro tears or full separation may occur under the stretch of the expanding uterus.

Without the stability of the linea alba anchoring them down, the two muscles of the rectus abdominis move further apart. This is most common in multiple pregnancies or after several pregnancies and with increasing age, and is called diastasis recti abdominis muscle (DRAM). The severity of this injury varies from mild (less than 3.5cm gap) to severe (more than 5cm gap). There are many really brilliant rehabilitative strategies and these are described in chapter 8, but the most significant thing to say here is that if we're not closed down the middle, then it makes sense that the front of our pelvis and our pelvic floor are not completely closed either. If the front door isn't shut then our home is not secure, so it's no wonder that those of us with DRAM are significantly more likely to experience back pain and pelvic floor dysfunction, including incontinence and pelvic organ prolapse, as well.

Side walls

Now you're becoming an expert in your own body you've probably already guessed that there is an inside and outside layer of muscles here! These are called the internal and external obliques. Running at an angle from our ribcage to our pelvis, one on top of the other, there is a left-sided internal and external oblique, and a separate right-sided pairing, and they blend with the front wall and the back wall just like in your house. As your obliques line your rib cage they can play a key role in repairing the 4cm overstretch around your bra straps caused by pregnancy, and restoring your ribcage circumference is key in tummy muscle recovery after pregnancy and birth.

These muscles are big and powerful, helping us to bend sideways, twist and flex our bodies. However, because they are big and powerful they can often become dominant, which means they can take over from the deeper transversus abdominis and rectus abdominis if they have been weakened in pregnancy. Therefore, we need to pay particular attention when rehabilitating our abdominal cylinder that we strengthen all four walls, both inside and out. If you can't wait, then tasks 12 to 15 (on pages 157–173) will take you through this process step by step.

Back yard

When we think of our tummy and pelvic floor strength, we often take the strength in our lower backs for granted. If we stick with our house analogy, the integrity and strength of the wall at the back are just as important as at the front, sides, top and bottom. Again, we have a deep muscle layer, our multifidus, and a superficial muscle layer. As a group these are called the erector spinae, which do what they say on the Latin tin and keep our spines erect. Our deep tummy muscles wrap around and connect with the multifidus at the back. Together with the pelvic floor and diaphragm they make up our primary sling, which is what we call this group of muscles that work together to give us strength enough for everyday function. With connections to every spinal disc and vertebrae, the multifidus keeps our backs strong and stable both through movement and when we are still. Changes in our shape and posture can make it harder for this muscle to do its job, but exercising it, like any muscle, rebuilds its strength regardless of these challenges. As this muscle is so deep it can be hard to feel its action. The best way to ensure it's working is exercising in spinal positions which we call 'neutral.' Too big a curve in our backs and the multifidus is pulled too tight to work. Too small a curve and the multifidus is stretched and lengthened, making it hard for it to contract and shorten. However, in a neutral spinal curve – not too big and not too flat – the multifidus muscles can shorten, contract, lengthen and stretch (tasks 1 and 2 on pages 30–39 cover exactly how to do this).

The erector spinae muscles are the big ones you can feel running all the way up your back either side of your spine. Place your hands here and when you move you will likely feel these muscles move too. Much like the multifidus, these muscles are happiest when you find a neutral spinal curve. With your hands either side of your spine and fingers pointing down towards your bottom, practise making a large curve in your lower back and then flattening it out, sticking out your bottom and then tucking it under. Notice that the muscles change, working harder and becoming tense when you arch, and softening and relaxing when you flatten out.

Now if we spend too long in either extreme, things can start to go wrong, not only here in the back, but throughout the entire abdominal cylinder. Too arched and the erector spinae muscles become tight, the joints in the back can pinch and become sore, and our tummy muscles can stretch. In this position our diaphragm and ribcage are open and stretched, and can feel weakened or difficult to close. You might notice that full breaths feel uncomfortable and your bras no longer fit around your ribcage. With our tails stuck out behind us our pelvic floor is pulled taut and often struggles to relax. When the curve is too flat the erector spinae become lazy and weak, and the joints in the back open up putting our spinal discs at risk of injury, while everything at the front – our tummy, inner thigh and pelvic floor – become lax or slack and hard to tighten. Our diaphragm and the muscles at our waist (our obliques) can become short, tight and dominant, overworking and causing pain and difficulty closing a tummy gap.

Clearly neither of these pictures sound great for healthy function and strength, but even worse, they challenge our whole system, right down to the messages our brain receives from our new body position and the adaptions the nerves make to accommodate this.

The control panel

Last but no means least, let's consider the control panel, both the buttons we can control and the ones we cannot – our nerve impulses. Our body's every action occurs as a result of a series of nerve impulses, which connect our brain, spinal cord and nerves to the muscles, joints and organs themselves. Our awareness of movement, pain or discomfort occurs via a series of nerve impulses travelling in the opposite direction – from the muscle, joint or organ to the spinal cord and up to the recognition centres in our brain. The nerves which run to and from our pelvis, pelvic floor and pelvic organs pass through the sacrum into the pelvis and line the pelvic floor and birth canal. Changes in our posture in pregnancy and motherhood can alter how these nerves send and receive messages. Pain, 'weakness', loss of sexual sensation or bladder and bowel control can all occur as a result of a misfiring in our wiring. This can last for just a few hours after birth, such as when the nerves in the birth canal are squashed by a baby's head, or, in the event of a bigger injury, much longer.

Just like the electrical wiring in our homes, re-wiring our body's nervous system can be a lengthy process, but it is possible. To do this you don't need an electrician or anyone else at all, you just need to practise what you want your body to do. Repeating the right movements and unlearning compensatory patterns will re-wire your system. Sending messages up and down the nerves from body part to brain and back again, and finding new pathways, is the medicine for this healing, which is why I cannot give you just one exercise to 'fix all'. However, taking on board all the tasks you find in this book, using what feels relevant and sticking to it, will re-write your body's messaging, and improve your strength and ultimately your function.

While synchronising all these anatomical aspects may seem daunting and too big a puzzle to rebuild, often it is just one part that holds the key to your healing and strength. Let's see what we can achieve.

TASK 1 FINDING THE FLOOR OF YOUR PELVIS

KIT YOU WILL NEED: A chair or gym ball.

If you can do this task sitting on a gym ball (one of those giant inflated balls often reserved for early labour), then this will give you the most contact with (and feedback from) your pelvic floor, but a firm chair will do just as well. A long mirror is also a good idea, so you can really see what's happening with your posture, and will give your body and brain more feedback than you can simply feel.

Start by rocking, tilting, tucking and untucking your pelvis, changing the shape in your lower back from a deep arch to a rounded curve. When you rock back, your tail will tuck right under. You will 'fall off' the sitting bones and on to your fleshy bottom and tail. Try to get far back onto your tailbone so that it goes underneath you. Then check out the rest of your posture! Your shoulders roll forwards and up, tightening your chest and stretching the muscles in the upper back. Your head pokes out, pinching your neck. Your tummy buckles and spills forwards, and your back muscles stretch.

Now correct your posture by reversing this movement, rocking forwards, off your tail and back up on to your sitting bones. Go further still and transfer all the weight on to your vulva and further still to the very front of your pelvis, your pubic bone. When you do this your chest opens up, your ribs flare forwards, your tummy and pelvic floor pull taut and your lower back pinches.

Get a feel for going between these two extreme positions, focusing on transferring your weight between the front and back of your pelvis. When you've got the hang of this, notice the changes in the rest of your body. Are you familiar with any of the pinch, stretch or buckling feelings or are these positions into which your body naturally falls? It's not just what you can see on the outside that's changing, but the muscles on the inside too. Where do you like to hang out? Where do you feel most comfortable? Just notice the shape of your curves – are they deep or shallow? Can you make out any curves or do you feel you're moving as one big block? Where do you like to sit? With your tail out back or tucked under? Don't try to change anything yet – just observe.

Next let's find the middle position, this lies halfway between the two extremes, with your pelvis and spine in *neutral*. Here your weight is shared evenly across the front, middle and tail of the pelvis. How easy is it to stay here? Is it natural or does it need some re-training?

Now find and touch with your fingers four points in turn; your pubis at the front, your left and right sitting bones underneath you, and your tailbone behind. Feel the contact between these four points and the chair or ball you are sitting on. Running underneath you between these four points is your pelvic floor. Keep feeling for these landmarks as you come back to rocking and rolling your pelvis. Notice how the bones come together as you rock backwards and part as you rock forwards, and how your sitting bones move apart when your tail is out and together when your tail is tucked under. The length and shape of the muscles running underneath and between these four points is changing too. The pelvic floor which attaches to these bones is widening and narrowing, shortening and lengthening. When your sitting bones and tail are stuck out your pelvic floor is long and taught. When your tail and sitting bones are tucked under it is slack and buckled. Come to the middle position, halfway between these two extremes, in neutral, and notice the tension is neither tight nor loose.

Next we're going to try to pull these four points together like the corners of a handkerchief; sitting bone to sitting bone, pubis to tail. As if your pelvic floor is the handkerchief slung between these points and you are picking it up from the middle, draw the edges and its four corners together. Keep your

31

bottom relaxed so that this feeling of gathering and lifting is inside your body. You can support this feeling with your hands if your body needs more feedback on what it should be doing. With your hand wrapping around your pubic bone on to your vulva, lift up everything you can feel with your hand as you tighten and pull the four corners of your imaginary handkerchief together, supporting the gathering and upward movement you want to feel on the inside with your hand on the outside. Try not to hold your breath or bring in any other muscles.

Now can you let it all go? Just as important as gathering the four corners of your handkerchief together is releasing them, allowing the muscles to retract back to their starting points, as you lie your handkerchief back down and spread it out flat. Just let it go and try not to push it down.

You don't need to hold this gather and lift of your pelvic floor at this point – just find it. Turn it all on, then let it all go. This action sends the signals from the brain down the nerve to the muscle and the muscle feeds back up the chain to tell the brain what's going on. Our first job is to restore this connection and control – the strength will come later.

When you get this right you may also notice your transversus abdominis contracting. You may be aware of an 'up and inward' feeling in your lower tummy. Or if you place your fingers at your knicker line you will likely feel this muscle press up against your fingers. The pelvic floor and transversus are connected, and once you've restored their connection through practise they will fire up together. Don't worry if you can't feel it, it doesn't mean it's not working. It's just that it's the deepest of all your muscles and is difficult to feel. It's worth mentioning here that the rest of your abdominal muscles should stay relaxed with this level of contraction. They will get their chance to re-train and work shortly, but this is all about the foundations.

Repeat this not only in the middle neutral pelvis position, but also with the pelvis rolled back, tail tucked under and your body slouched, and then with your pelvis rolled forward and tail out. Hopefully you can feel that the two extremes make this action harder to perform. You will probably find this exercise easiest in neutral.

Practise this where you spend much of your time – at your desk, in the car or standing. What's your default position? Let's restore, rebuild and retrain in neutral instead.

What's important

- Healing and rebuilding after pregnancy and having a baby is a 'whole body' mission.
- The pelvis is the base of the spine and the connecting point between the upper and lower body. All our movements pass through here. When you move your pelvis, you move your pelvic floor. When healing and rebuilding the floor, you must also consider the walls and the roof.
- The pelvic floor is quite literally the floor of the pelvis. The abdominal muscles and spinal muscles are the walls. The diaphragm is the roof. Figuring out how to fix the pelvic floor means looking at everything, including the walls and the roof.
- The diaphragm, tummy, back and pelvic floor muscles work as one unit. When you're trying to get strong again you need to think about all four – and restore the brain, nerve muscle connections of each individually and together.
- In spinal neutral, all of our muscles work at their best. Check your posture and find your curves.

2. Posture: Strike a pose

When women come to see me for pain, pelvic floor problems or tummy muscle separation, posture is one of the first things they mention. They admit, 'My posture isn't great,' disheartteningly resigned to this fact, certain that it cannot be changed, but the reality is that with a few simple exercises peppered throughout your day it can be. And it's important: our posture is everything. To build a comfortable home for ourselves we need secure foundations and dependable scaffolding (our bony skeleton) on which to lay our high-quality building materials (our muscles). When our bones, muscles and nervous system are all working, pulling and pushing together, we achieve the perfect balance – the ability to maintain a relatively stable state despite changes in the world outside. Our posture is both a consequence and a reflection of our strength. If we change the muscles, we move the scaffolding, and our frame and consequently our shape alters too. If we move the scaffolding and change our shape, we affect our muscle length and strength. The result of these changes shows in our posture.

Instead of 'My posture *isn't* great,' try 'My posture *wasn't* great.' Decide to make the change and have confidence in your ability to reach the goal. New mothers often tell me their postural differences are due to many hours spent feeding and cradling their newborn baby, so this is one of the first things we tackle.

Mastering breastfeeding, bottle feeding and nursing a baby with reflux are huge feats in their own right, even more so if you're entertaining a toddler at the same time. Doing these things with the best posture may seem one ask too many, but it will serve both of you. When you sit more comfortably your baby will too. When you feel more relaxed and in less discomfort you will be able to nurse your baby or maybe even simultaneously read to your toddler with more ease. It is worth the time to set yourself up and ask others to help you to do this too.

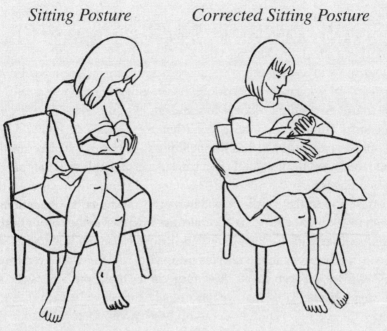

Sitting Posture *Corrected Sitting Posture*

How to sit and feed your baby

If you can recognise the first posture you will probably relate to the tightness building in your mid-back as you twist. This can be aggravated by the weight of your baby in your arms, and can result in neck and back pain. When we cross our legs like this the back of our pelvis opens and stretches, and can pinch painfully at the front.

Instead, shuffle your bottom to the back of the chair. If your back isn't fully supported then stick a pillow behind you. Hold a Pilates ball or cushion between your knees to stop you crossing your legs, but also to fire up your inner thigh and pelvic floor (bonus!). Use as many pillows as you need to lift your baby to your breast or bottle. Often one feeding pillow isn't enough and you may need a pillow from your bed underneath this to get the right height. Your baby should feel fully supported without your hands needing to hold them, leaving you free to hold the bottle, lift your nipple to their nose or simply caress your baby as they feed.

To improve our posture we must stretch what is tight, strengthen what is long and loosen what is stiff. Sounds complicated? Thankfully, I've broken rebuilding our posture down into two uncomplicated tasks, but first we need to work out which one best fits you.

Imagine you're building your home from scratch. The most important part is where you lay its foundations, because these need to be strong, stable and secure. Now think of these foundations as your pelvis, the very base of your torso. How we hold our pelvis when we're sitting or standing dictates our spinal position above. Just like building your house, the placement of the foundations and the first few bricks you lay will dictate how strong and stable the building is.

Unlike the straight walls of our homes, we were built with four natural curves in our back. Our spine naturally has extended arches at our necks and lower backs, rounded curves in our mid-backs and at our tailbone. Designed for shock absorption and to take the pressure off the individual vertebrae and the soft discs between them, these four curves make our spines the strong and capable scaffolding that we rely on, allowing us to bend and flex. If we change the shape, position or depth of these curves, then we change the co-ordination, timing and strength of our muscular walls and we might find it harder to bend, flex or absorb everyday loads. This can make the movement we take for granted in our daily lives more effortful and even painful.

'Sway back' posture is typical for the mums I see in my clinic. When we roll our pelvis backwards, tuck under our tail and slouch, we flatten out the natural arch in our lower back, opening up the joints of the pelvis and 'unlocking' our sacrum. Our sacrum (the bone right at the bottom of our backs, tucked inside our knickers) is often seen as the keystone by physios – like that one important brick at the top of a stone archway. If we move this keystone, the archway collapses. When we unlock our sacrum our ribcage sinks downwards and our spine takes on a C curve from top to bottom, jutting our heads and shoulders forwards. This position puts strain on our spinal muscles and its discs, and buckles the tummy muscles and pelvic floor. In this posture we women, and new mothers particularly, become susceptible to a rather terrifying shopping list of disc injury, pelvic ligament pain, pelvic floor weakness, pelvic organ prolapse and tummy muscle separation. But do not fear – we're learning what can go wrong so that we can fix it, starting with your foundations and rebuilding the scaffolding and brickwork on top.

When we stand in sway back our bottom muscles are doing nothing; they are lax and 'switched off'. The hamstrings are short and tight in this position, while the front of the legs are long and stretched, creating a 'flat bottom'. The muscles at our sides will be dominant, short and tight, but our horizontal corset muscles are left long and lax. We've tucked our tail underneath us, moving it further towards the pubic bone. The pelvic floor hammock which is slung between these two bones is loose and slack, making it much harder to find and ultimately strengthen.

But perhaps you can relate to the opposite? If we roll our pelvis forwards and exaggerate our lumbar arch, our sacrum, its tail and consequently our bottom sticks out behind us, pert and prominent like a Kardashian's. The back of our pelvis and its keystone is now pinched closed and compressed, making this vulnerable to pain. With our abdominal strength compromised at the front through pregnancy and after giving birth, and with the keystone displaced at the back, the front of our pelvis is also now vulnerable. The joint here can open up, stretching our tummies and the pelvic floor, which attaches to it, even further. Making up for the generous extension and inward curve at the bottom of our spine, the upper back flexes and rounds forwards in an attempt to re-centre our weight. Unless we stay looking at our toes, we now have to over-arch our neck to face front and bring the head back on to our shoulders! Unsurprisingly this puts a lot of strain on the joints of the back and the muscles which attach to it. In this posture our abdominal wall is long and stretched, and the back muscles are short and tight. The back of the legs (hamstrings) are long and stretched, while the hip flexors at the front are shortened and tightened, pulling the pelvis forwards. These changes lengthen and stretch our pelvic floor, making it harder to contract, shorten and tighten. Because the inward curve of the spine is called a lordosis, this is known as lordotic posture. In this position we are susceptible to tummy muscle separation, pelvic floor injury, bladder weakness, and pain at the pubic symphysis and in our lower backs. This might not sound like an attractive option either, but there is a third way.

Our optimal posture is somewhere between these two extremes, with four clear curves in our back. In this position our pelvis, secured by our keystone sacrum, provides the most stable base for our spinal vertebrae and the discs stacked on top. The muscles of our abdominal cylinder have perfect resting tension; not too loose, not too tight. This is our *neutral spinal posture*. We all started here, before pregnancy, work or sport changed the way we sit and stand, but getting back there is possible. To correct either posture, we need to address these muscular imbalances; to stretch what is tight and strengthen what is long.

I've met many women who have consciously tried to avoid the lordotic 'big-bottomed' Kardashian posture and instead have been tucking their bottoms under to try to shrink their tummies and behinds, and misguidedly 'protect' their backs and pelvic floors. Their minds are blown when I show them this simple towel trick and their posture instantly changes to a more neutral, middle ground. Try it now…

Run a towel or scarf underneath your pelvis from your pubic bone at the front to your tail at the back. Now imagine this fabric is the pelvic floor hammock slung between your legs and connecting to these two bones. Notice the changes in shape and tension in the fabric as you move your bones and change your posture. With your tail tucked underneath you towards the pubic bone the fabric becomes slack. Here we are much more likely to suffer from low tone pelvic floor conditions such as not being able to hold a full bladder, leaking urine and pelvic organ prolapse. Do the opposite: stick your tail and bottom out behind you and the fabric becomes tense and taut. Here you are much more likely to experience symptoms of a pelvic floor that struggles to relax, including pain, dribbling urine and not fully emptying your bladder or bowel. Come back to neutral and the pelvic floor is just right; not too tight and not too lax, able to lift and release, as are the muscles of the entire abdominal cylinder. To get here and stay here we need to address the tug of war between the front and back of the body.

You can see that wherever the bony pelvis and its keystone sits dictates the position of our spine, our ribcage and everything else above. And it is not just our skeleton that has changed shape, but our muscles too. It is our muscles that have made us move. The strength, tone and tension of our muscles have just as much a say, if not more, in the position of our bony scaffolding as the bones themselves. Like trying to touch our toes, if the back of our legs are tight we blame our hamstrings for this inflexibility, but if we release our tail and allow our hamstrings to let go and bottom stick out, look how much further the muscles can stretch!

Pregnancy and birth, as well as sitting hunched over a computer, playing sports and repetitive tasks can all lead to changes in our posture. Real postural strength is varied and changes as much as we do, keeping our joints stable and secure when we're sitting, bending, walking, carrying a toddler, in pregnancy and in birth. What we want is for our pelvis and its keystone to comfortably twist, open and close, and still find its way back to neutral. Similarly, we want our spines to bend, flex, extend, twist and combine all these movements together, as well as becoming straight and finding its curves once more. These are all naturally occurring shape changes that our bodies are capable of and that we can do with 'normal' muscle function. But when there is pain, muscle weakness or injury, these everyday movements can become problematic and our posture gradually changes. Let's find our way back to where we started.

TASK 2 STANDING TALLER, LIVING STRONGER

To work out which path to follow stand against a wall, rest your back and bottom here and take one step forwards. With a small bend in your knees you should feel supported by the wall. Now use your hand to find the top of your bottom, where your sacrum meets the rest of the spine. Can you slide your hand easily under here? Is there a large gap between you and the wall? Yes? You are likely to be in 'lordotic posture'. Follow this route to stretch and strengthen. Or is there no room for your hand to slide. Is your lower back and sacrum glued to the wall? Yes? You are likely to be in sway back posture. Follow these tasks to make your way back to neutral.

IF YOU HAVE LORDOTIC POSTURE

Your checklist of exercises includes: *loosening up* your lower back; *stretching* the front of your thighs and your spinal muscles; and *strengthening* your tummy muscles and hamstrings.

KIT YOU WILL NEED: A chair, sofa or big gym ball.

Spinal mobility:

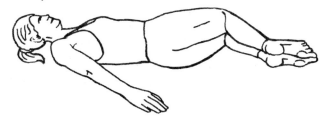

39

This feels like wiggling a cork free from a bottle of wine. Lying on your back with your knees bent, squeeze your legs together and roll your knees over to one side, allowing your bottom and lower back to lift, while keeping your shoulder blades firmly on the ground. Squeeze your legs together as you roll your legs back to the middle, then over to the opposite side. As you roll from side to side notice any tightness in your back free up, just like loosening that cork! Work from side to side for 2-4 minutes.

Thigh stretch:

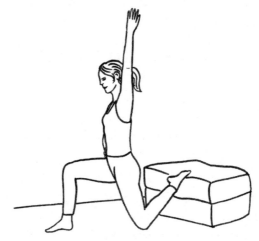

You will need the chair for this one. Take a few steps away from the chair then reach one leg backwards. Bend your front knee and push your hips forwards, tucking your tail underneath you. If you are using the edge of a sofa or low chair you can lower all the way down to the ground and hold it here. At the same time create length in your back by imagining your head is a helium balloon floating up towards the ceiling. You should feel the stretch in the front of the back thigh. Take the back arm up to the sky to deepen the stretch and lift from your breastbone, as though you have a shiny necklace on that you want to show off to the room. Hold for 30 seconds. Repeat x2 on each side.

Childs pose:

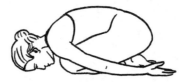

On your hands and knees, drop your chin to your chest, round your spine, look into your belly button and tuck your tail underneath you, stretching your whole back line. Next push your weight back to rest your bottom on your heels. Keep your arms reaching forward for the deepest stretch or bring them by your side. Hold it here for 1 minute, release back to all fours then repeat.

Hamstring bridge:

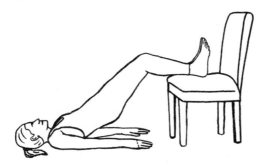

Lying on the floor raise your feet up onto the edge of the chair or sofa. Lift your hips up, pressing down through your feet until there is a straight line from your knees through to your hips and shoulders. You want the back of your legs to be working here, much more than the muscles in your back. Watch out for your ribs flaring forwards, keep them tucked in, and try not to push the chair or sofa away. Next bend at your hips, lowering your bottom to the floor and repeat x20. Rest for 10 seconds. Repeat x3.

Tummy muscle strengthening:

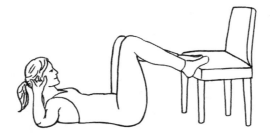

Lie with your legs supported on your chair or sofa so that the front of your hips stay relaxed. Now press your lower back into the floor so that your tummy button pulls in. As you breathe out lift your head and shoulders up towards the ceiling, not down towards your knees. This part is very important to prevent downward pressure on the pelvic floor. Imagine your head and shoulders are a drawer being pulled from your body, the dresser, towards the ceiling. Your tummy should pull in flatter, not bulge outwards. If it bulges then come back to this one once you've completed chapter 8. Hold and breathe for 10 seconds. Lower. Repeat x6.

IF YOU HAVE SWAY BACK POSTURE

Your checklist of exercises includes: *loosening up* your feet and pelvic ligaments; *stretching* your hamstrings and chest; and *strengthening* your bottom and back muscles.

KIT YOU WILL NEED: A massage ball. Also known as a lacrosse or trigger point ball, this firm rubber sphere can massage and stretch tissues, just as a traditional hands-on massage would. You can work it into muscles and ligaments with your hands or lean, roll and lie on it to relieve pain from knotted and tense tissues all across the body. We will use this tool here and in the tasks that follow to relax contracted muscles, help circulation and blood flow, and stimulate muscle stretch reflexes. This means less pain, more flexibility.

Foot release: The feet often house a whole lot of tension, so this is absolute magic! A foot massage releases the legs, hips, back and pelvis, and don't worry if you don't have anyone on hand to do this for you, because one of the best tools in our physio kit is a massage ball. Stand and press the ball of your foot down on the massage ball, pressing and releasing repeatedly for 30 seconds. Then move the ball to the arch of your foot, pressing and releasing for 30 seconds. Finish by pressing your foot on to the ball and rolling it forwards and backwards, fanning out your toes as you go, again for 30 seconds.

Pelvic ligament release: This is just as orgasmic as the foot release! You're trying to trace the arc of the sacro-tuberus and sacro-iliac ligaments across each side of your bottom (see page 20 for a recap on where to find these). Start up against a wall with the ball near your sitting bone and lean into it. Bend your knees to slide down the wall allowing the ball to move up and in towards the edge of your sacrum. Continue to roll up and down, staying on any tender spots until they release, for up to 60 seconds. Do both sides, one may be more tender or need more work than the other. If it's too tender to start with, try the foot release first – it's amazing how releasing your feet affects everything higher up so quickly.

Hamstring stretch:

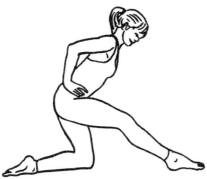

The tug of war on the pelvic bones is often fought between the hamstring muscles at the back of the thigh and the hip flexors at the front. Start in kneeling and step one leg out in front of you. In this position you can alternate between stretching the front and the back of your thigh. Keeping your back straight, hinge forwards from your hips and push your seat back. Maybe even reach around behind you with your hand and lift your bottom cheek up. Keep your front leg straight to feel a stretch down the back of your leg and sink your body down to it as though you're going to give your knee a kiss. Hold for 30 seconds then release back to centre and lean your body backwards. Push your back hip forwards to feel a stretch now at the front of the back leg. Simultaneously squeeze your elbows together behind you to open and stretch your chest. Imagine you are wearing a gorgeous necklace and want to show it off – lift your breastbone up to the sun, so that the light bounces off your necklace. Hold for 30 seconds. Repeat x2 before changing sides.

Bottom activation:

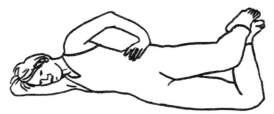

Lying on your side, bend your knees so that your feet stick out behind you (off the mat if you're using one). Lift both of your feet off the floor to roll your pelvis forwards. Now open your top knee and press your heels firmly together. You should feel the squeeze working in both bottom cheeks. Hold this for 30 seconds x4 on each side.

Lower back strengthening: Lying on your tummy, bend your legs like a frog – with your knees wide but your feet together – and firmly press your heels together. You will feel your back and bottom activate as these muscles tighten and close your pelvis. You can always reach around to your lower back here to check these muscles are responding as they should! Hold for 10 seconds. Release. Repeat x6.

What's important

- Rather than an afterthought, postural changes are a crucial step to feeling stronger.

- Posture is both a reflection and a result of our strength.

- When you're sitting, imagine your head is a helium balloon, floating up towards the ceiling and pulling your entire body with it. Roll your weight on to the middle of your pelvis rather than all on to your tail.

- When you're standing, think of your favourite necklace or even put it on. Now show it off, let the light bounce off it and notice how you stand taller, drop your shoulders and relax into it.

- Make whatever you're carrying – a bag, a baby or a toddler – part of you. Hold it close to your body and let your head float skywards, show off your necklace and grow stronger in this position with what you're carrying as close to the centre of your body as possible. Backpacks and carriers, wheelie bags and buggies all provide better solutions to carrying than lopsided on one arm.

3. The pelvic floor: You didn't know how good it was until it wasn't

The pelvic floor has long been a mythical creature for many women, whose powers and strength they cannot trust or believe in. I have found that little thought is given to this part of our body until it starts playing up. Sadly, pelvic floor complaints such as wetting our knickers and parping in public are far too common after pregnancy and birth. But while they are common, that doesn't mean they are normal, nor does it mean we should hide, put up with or manage these symptoms on our own. So how do you know when your pelvic floor is not working properly? Here are some of the symptoms you may notice:

- Leaking urine with forceful activities (for example, laughing or sneezing). This is known as 'stress incontinence'.
- An urgent need to go for a wee and perhaps not making it in time. This is called 'urge incontinence'.
- A combination of stress and urge incontinence. This is known as 'mixed incontinence'.
- Incomplete bladder emptying.
- Bowel urgency or incontinence.
- Incomplete bowel emptying, struggling to go, hard stools and constipation.
- Wind escaping accidently or farting in public without warning. This is known as 'flatus incontinence', 'vaginal flatulence' or fanny farts (although I much prefer the term 'queefing').
- Getting up in the night to pee or wetting the bed.
- Vulva, vaginal, bladder, urethra, or pelvic pain, respectively called 'vulvodynia', 'vaginismus', 'interstitial cystitis' and 'pelvic pain syndrome'.
- Reduced sexual desire, sensation or orgasms, or lack of arousal and pain.

- Heaviness, bulging into the vagina, laxity, too much movement or a sense of everything falling out – in other words the symptoms of prolapse. Its full and official name is 'pelvic organ prolapse' which is often abbreviated to POP (and you may well feel that things have popped out).

It's amazing how many of us will put up with these symptoms and even start to regard them as normal, but the emotional costs of coping with these injuries can be huge. It's not surprising that post-pregnancy pelvic floor problems are closely linked to feelings of low self-esteem, poor quality of life and even post-natal depression. This can have a huge impact on our lives and relationships, stopping us from living as we choose. While we know incontinence and prolapse are associated with feeling ashamed, embarrassed and even depressed, we often suffer this fight in silence. But we don't need to put up with this. It is not OK. We can change this and you can feel better. Read on for the tools and support you need to recover and start to leave these problems in the past.

It's important for me to say here that while I have put all I know and can share with you into this book, it is not, of course completely tailored to you. If you feel that you need more of an individualised approach then a physical assessment with a women's health physiotherapist is the best place to start. Make an appointment with your GP, share your concerns and ask to be referred for physiotherapy. If the waiting list is too long and you can afford it, you can make an appointment directly. Go to thepogp.co.uk to find registered private and NHS women's health physios in your area. Your first appointment will take up to one hour and sometimes this is all you need – to be fully assessed, taught how to do the relevant exercises correctly and then sent on your way to practise them and feel stronger.

What and where is the pelvic floor?

As we now know, it is the floor of our pelvis, the ground floor of our home and a hammock for our pelvic organs. As you work through these next sections you're going to dig a bit deeper than this and you're going to get to know all its beautiful parts intimately. You're going to feel each muscle working, from the lips of your vulva to the neck of your womb, isolating and engaging the muscles which make up your back passage, vaginal wall and bladder mechanism, pinching, lifting, squeezing but above all controlling them.

Throughout your body there are two types of muscle fibres: fast twitch – the ones responsible for big explosive movements; and slow twitch – these have less force, but are great for endurance and maintaining strength over a longer period of time. Our pelvic floor muscles are 70% slow twitch fibres. This means that in theory they have great endurance and you are unlikely to feel the same post-exercise muscle soreness you experience after lifting heavy weights.

When we think of our pelvic floor we might think of the muscles which stop us peeing, but although there are muscles here, there is also a whole web of intricately connected muscles deeper inside, filling our pelvis with muscular layers from hip to hip and back to front.

Let's start with the superficial layer of muscles, which you're probably most familiar with: your urethral sphincter, anal sphincter and bulbospongiosus. OK, so their names might sound obscure and more like comic book villains,

The Pelvic Floor

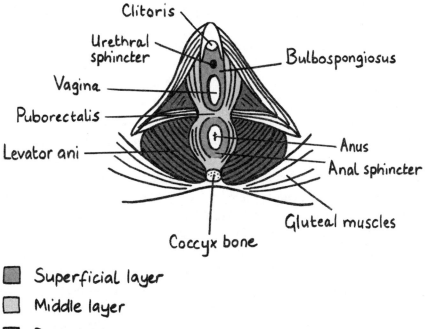

Clitoris

Urethral sphincter

Vagina

Puborectalis

Levator ani

Bulbospongiosus

Anus

Anal sphincter

Gluteal muscles

Coccyx bone

■ Superficial layer
□ Middle layer
■ Deep layer

but you work with these guys on a daily basis. These circular rings of muscles sit where our wee, poo and vaginal canals meet the outside of our body, to clench, pinch and tighten these outlets. Their action is controlled both sub-consciously and consciously, meaning they work without us telling them to and also when we ask them to. They stop wee and poo from escaping throughout the day, but we can clench them on demand as well, including the bulbospongiosus (you really do have one – part the lips of your vagina to see your vaginal opening and there it is).

The middle layer of your pelvic floor muscles – the puborectalis – runs from your pubic bone at the front to your tail at the back, wrapping around each of your pelvic outlets. This is a pretty awesome muscle which can kink the wee, poo and vaginal pipes in the same way that kinking a hosepipe stops the flow. Again, it works well with little conscious effort from us until we need it to work harder, such as when our bladder is full to bursting and we're in a queue for the loo or when we feel the need to break wind in an inappropriate place. Then it lifts and tightens further and even presses the urethra against the pubic bone to ensure nothing can escape.

The deepest layer of muscle is the levator ani. This is a big span of individual muscles called the pubococcygeus, iliococcygeus and coccygeus. Their job is to pull the entire pelvic ring together and lift the bladder, womb and bowel higher into the pelvis. The levator ani may feel out of reach and the hardest to find consciously, and I often find it is left out of pelvic floor exercises, but it is honestly possible to work this muscle on demand too.

While we can only see the most superficial of the pelvic floor muscles from the outside, we can feel the deeper layers by inserting a finger into the vagina or back passage. Women's and men's physios examine the pelvic floor muscles in this way. In fact, if you've ever been examined by a women's health physiotherapist you may recall being given your strength as a number, a bit like a score card. We assess all muscles on their strength, according to the Oxford scale. This was modified for the pelvic floor by a brilliant physio called Jo Laycock. Using this 0 to 5 scale and one or two fingers inside the vaginal canal pressing into the muscles, we can objectively measure your strength baseline and track your improvements. You can check your strength yourself if you feel comfortable, but don't worry if you can't plot yourself accurately on the scale, you are just checking for improvements and feeling a stronger contraction as you work through the rehabilitation tasks. Here's what you might feel:

(5) Strong: When you press against it there's a strong squeeze and lift or kink of your finger. You can also lift bit by bit and release bit by bit, hold the contraction as long as you want, pulse it, pause it, play a tune…(that last one's a joke!)

(4) Good contraction with a lift: There is enough muscle here to create a squeeze and lift your finger. You need a strength of (4) or (5) to protect against a prolapse.

(3) Moderate contraction: The muscle is working, but it isn't quite strong enough to lift your finger.

(2) Weak, inconsistent contraction: The muscles aren't working together to create a strong enough squeeze.

(1) Flicker: Something's happening, the signal is getting through, but it's not enough to create a contraction yet.

(0) Nothing: In cases where the nerve to the muscle has been injured in some way you may feel nothing when you send those messages from your brain to your pelvic floor. Don't panic if you feel nothing. It may just be that you're not feeling in quite the right places. Ask a physiotherapist, doctor or midwife to check for you in the first instance.

A word of caution though: it's not all about the number, but more about our muscles' ability to work together from a stable skeletal base; to feel everything both contract and relax completely. We often focus on the pelvic floor tightening and lifting, but less so on the muscles releasing and letting go. When you consider the pelvic floor's function, this releasing action is just as – if not more – important than the strengthening. When our pelvic floor muscles are not working together a range of problems, such as those outlined above can occur. And we cannot ignore the emotional impact that these have on our self-esteem, body image and mental wellbeing.

The belief that these symptoms arise from pelvic floor muscle weakness alone is a common misconception. I regularly hear 'Kegels don't work' or 'I tried pelvic floor exercises but got nowhere' and 'I've been squeezing my muscles like I'm supposed to, but things feel worse.' Here's why: in order for the pelvic floor muscles to pull the pelvic ring closed, lift the pelvic organs and kink the pee and poo pipes to keep us continent and symptom-free, we need more than just Kegels. We need:

- The pelvis bones sitting in their most stable position.
- The pelvic organs sitting high enough up in the first place.
- A good nerve-to-muscle connection (nerves often can't carry the right messages when they are squashed by a baby's head or blurred with pain).
- Enough pelvic floor muscle fibres (the more muscle fibres, the stronger the muscle).
- Muscles which can both contract and relax... If they cannot relax not only will our bladder and bowel not empty fully, but we also can't create a strong enough lift. You can't lift, tense or contract something that is already lifted, tensed or contracted.

Most pelvic floor symptoms arise when the pelvic floor is too lax or too tense. We need to be on the lookout for an imbalance of some kind. Of the women who come to see me, 99% confidently tell me their pelvic floor is 'weak'. They are often stunned when I tell them it's actually the opposite. In fact, I see a 50:50 split between pelvic floors which are too weak and those which have become too tense following injury, trauma or pain. So how can one tell the difference?

Is my pelvic floor too lax?

The whole or part of the pelvic floor can become too lax when there is:

- A disconnect between the nerve and muscle so that the contraction cannot get through. This can happen in the long second stage of delivery when the baby's head presses on the pelvic floor nerves inside the birth canal, numbing their sensation or action, or when there has been a manual intervention in the delivery, such as ventouse or forceps, following trauma, abuse or surgery.
- Pelvic ring instability, when the bones and their ligaments are moving too much, so that the muscles attaching to them cannot stabilise and tighten. Those of us who are mobile and stretchy by nature will be more susceptible to our pelvis and pelvic floor stretching too much.
- An overstretch of the muscles and tendons beyond what they can tolerate. Like pulling an elastic band, the pelvic floor muscles can accommodate a stretch of up to three times their length. Beyond this, overstretch occurs

and, just as with an elastic band, they will struggle to return to their previous length. Traumatic births which involve ventouse, forceps, manual force or result in cuts or tears are all examples of the pelvic floor being stretched past what it can tolerate.

- A reduction in the amount of muscle bulk through lack of training, injury, strain or hormonal changes. Pregnancy is a perfect example of all of these factors!

To make it worse, these features often occur together. Particularly after pregnancy, which naturally alters our pelvic ring position and stability, and is then quickly followed by birth (vaginal or abdominal), which further stretches our muscles and joints. Consequently, the nerve to muscle connection is disrupted, our muscles cannot be accessed, activated or strengthened, and therefore our muscle bulk reduces. Inevitably the kinking mechanism of the pelvic floor muscle may not be enough to stop the passage of wee, wind or poo – oh joy! The kink and lift may become more of a soft bend, so that we can stem the flow, but not stop it all together. In addition, an overstretch of the soft tissues and the effects of gravity mean that the bladder, womb, bowel and their passages may not be sitting where they were previously. If they drop down into the vaginal space, as in prolapse, then the kinking and lifting action will need to be re-educated and made so much stronger than it was before to achieve the same result (more on this in chapter 6).

Symptoms of a pelvic floor which is too lax include:

Stress urinary incontinence: Leaking urine with activities the pelvic floor is not strong enough to withstand (even laughing can be a challenge too far after injury).

Urge incontinence: Urgency to go for a wee, poo or parp and perhaps not making it in time.

Sexual dysfunction: Reduced sensation, lack of arousal or orgasms.

Pelvic organ prolapse: Displacement of the pelvic organs and their pipes from their original position.

If you are experiencing any (or all!) of these symptoms, please don't despair. We must not consider these symptoms as normal, to be expected and put up with them. They are harm or physical trauma to our bodies and like all injuries they can take many forms. Our recovery can be straightforward and quick, or lengthy and complicated, but recovery is achievable. Injury can happen anywhere in the body and can be healed and rebuilt. Why should we think of injuries related to pregnancy and birth any differently because they are hidden in our underwear? I will teach you how to heal and rebuild in the following tasks.

Is my pelvic floor too tense?

Part of or the whole pelvic floor can become too tense when:

- There is pain present and the muscles are subconsciously guarding, protecting or compensating for this. This pain may not just be in the pelvic floor, but may also be in the back, hips or pelvis – as we now know, it's all connected.

- Following physical trauma such as birth tears and cuts. While the muscle is healing the body lays down more tissue than it needs to protect and rebuild. Over time and through massage, stretching and strengthening, the muscle remodels and tone, strength and function return.

- When weakness in one muscle is over-compensated for by tightness in another muscle, which is common after an episiotomy or perineal tear in childbirth. The pelvic floor is a multi-layered group of muscles, so if the muscle around the episiotomy site has been compromised and weakened, the muscle on the opposite side, the one that hasn't been cut or torn, may be trying to be helpful, overworking and becoming very tense as a result.

- Following psychological trauma, including periods of prolonged or acute stress. We humans (men included) can carry our stress in our most intimate and vulnerable of places. If you think of someone who's feeling stressed, you might notice their shoulders up by their ears. Now doing this without everything else moving up too feels impossible. Even the pelvic floor follows, becoming tense and contracted in this new position. Maybe your birth story is having a similar physical effect. Post-traumatic stress disorder (PTSD) following a difficult birth is a very real thing and is diagnosed in 9% of us after childbirth. Or maybe you're disappointed that your birth didn't go the way you planned. Regaining free movement in muscles that are so intimately connected to these feelings can be hard, but it is possible and essential to the healing of our body and mind.

Symptoms of a pelvic floor that is too tense include:

Stress urinary incontinence: Leaking urine during strenuous activities such as laughing, coughing, sneezing, running, jumping etc. When the pelvic floor is already tense and we increase the strain, asking it to do more, it can't – it has no more tensing to offer.

Incomplete emptying of the bladder: Think of maintaining a constant kink in a hosepipe – the water becomes trapped and won't flow freely.

Painful toileting, intercourse or even everyday movement: Just like when your neck is tense, you become conscious of the movements you make, and they can feel restricted and painful until the muscle releases again.

Incomplete bowel emptying, struggling to go or straining for a poo: These are all signs of constipation – if we cannot fully relax our muscles our bowel struggles to fully empty.

Getting up to pee or bed wetting: Both of these can happen when you relax in your sleep if you have not fully emptied your bladder in the daytime.

When you suspect your pelvic floor is too tense it can be beneficial to engage in whole-body movement and relaxation (I give you a head start on this in task 3 on page 55). Yoga is a great way to stretch through the pelvic floor and let it go, connecting your body and mind to release and relax. Heartbeat-raising exercise that leaves you breathless and sweaty is another way of creating a stretch and improving blood flow to the pelvic floor, feeding it with what it needs to heal and restore itself.

Women's health physiotherapists can also manually release the tense and overworked muscles of the pelvic floor, just like any other muscle in the body. Think of it as an internal massage. We manually stretch the tight muscles so that subsequent strengthening is more even and complete. We can teach you how to do this yourself and it can be as simple as inserting a (clean!) finger into your own vagina and pressing down until you feel a stretch, or we can employ wands or dilators if this feels easier for you. These massage tools are often made of smooth silicone and specifically designed to release hard-to-reach internal pelvic floor muscles.

Sometimes internal release can be too intense, bringing back difficult emotions and feel frightening or too invasive. This is OK. You will be OK. You do not have to endure or 'get through this'. There are other options. I encourage you to speak up and accept only what feels right and good for you, and to reject what doesn't. We can release and relax a tense or traumatised pelvic floor in other ways. Not all of us who have experienced neck pain and stiffness have required physiotherapy, but we've managed to work it out ourselves with exercise, relaxation and a little TLC. We can release the internal pelvic floor muscles by releasing its next-door neighbours, the muscles on the outside in our bottom, thighs, back, tummy and groin. Task 3 is all about stretching these external muscles and gently massaging out any tension, as this may be all that is needed to 'let go' internally.

So how do you know if your pelvic floor is too lax or too tense? Unfortunately it's not that black and white. Our pelvic floor can be both lax and tense all at the same time as it's made up of so many different parts. Not only this, but tone in our pelvic floor is as dynamic as we are. Its position and therefore tension changes all the time. The solution is to work the muscles through-range, which means completely contracting and completely relaxing them. If we always start with some stretching and relaxation, we can achieve more with our strengthening exercises. If we find that we were relaxed and loose already, then nothing is lost and no harm is done. We will just have greater awareness of where our muscles are and what they are doing.

Pelvic floor exercises

STEP 1

We need our pelvic floors to be strong and taut enough to support our pelvic organs, but also to be able to release and ease off enough for going to the loo, sex and birth. It's a tall order! However, it's achievable when we take things step by step. A pelvic floor that is already working too hard won't respond to your pelvic floor exercises as you imagined it would. If the pelvic floor is too tense to begin with you may struggle to tighten it any further, feel any lift at all, let alone reach your 'top level' contraction. You may already be there, working maximally just to keep upright, and the pelvic floor is not capable of squeezing, lifting or tightening any higher. First let's get back to the starting line so that you have a fair chance of succeeding in rebuilding.

▰▰TASK 3 LET IT GO

KIT YOU WILL NEED: A massage ball, although you could also use a spikey tumble dryer ball or golf ball if you don't have one.

Pelvic floor release with a ball: This is a great way to get your pelvic floor to relax. The internal pelvic floor muscles are next-door neighbors to our external bottom muscles, so if we release one we can release the other. Lying down, place a ball on the edge of your bony sacrum in your bottom, where it starts to get fleshy and where it might feel tender and tense. Try to relax down on to the ball so that your weight creates the pressure. There may be discomfort here and even create sensations which radiate out to other parts of your body. It may be enough to just hold it and allow those sensations to settle and come back to the ball. If you can't feel anything hug that leg up towards you so that you create a stretch at the same time. Hold this until the pressure or intensity eases, for up to 90 seconds, then move the ball up, down or out to find another spot of tension. Repeat up to four times on each side.

Puppy dog stretch:

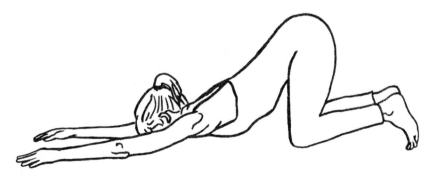

From all fours stick your bottom out behind you and lower your chest to the ground. Reach your arms forward and if you can, rest your forehead on the ground. In this position think about sticking your 'tail' in the air while your chest sinks down to your mat, just like a puppy playing chase. Imagine a diamond at your seat running between your tail and your pubic bone, and your sitting bones at either bottom crease. Try to make this diamond as open as possible, stretching it wider as you sink deeper. Locate the sitting bones in your bottom creases and try to stretch them away from one another, so that your whole seat relaxes. Hold and breathe for 1-2 minutes or until you feel relaxed.

Happy baby:

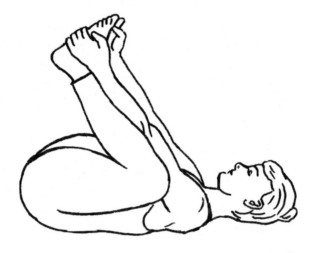

You can do this with one leg or with both at the same time, whichever feels most comfortable for you. Lying on your back pull one or both knees towards your shoulders. Reach down between your legs to take a hold of one or both feet. Allow your knees to drop down towards your shoulder blades and gently stretch your feet apart. For a deeper stretch keep hold of your feet and straighten your legs while keeping your knees close to your chest. You'll feel a stretch down the back of your legs, on your inner thighs and across your pelvic floor. Hold for 1–2 minutes or until you feel relaxed.

If you are prone to pelvic floor pain, identify with pelvic floor tightness or just struggle to let go, it's a good idea to repeat this task each time you do your pelvic floor muscle strengthening exercise or just when you need to restore resting tone to prevent the pelvic floor becoming tense again. You're looking for a clear difference between feeling 'contracted' and 'relaxed'.

STEP 2

Okay we're relaxed and ready to go, so let's get to the pelvic floor exercises. A disruption between the nerve and muscle is really common and quite normal in pregnancy and birth. No matter how long ago these events took place, you need to check in with your nerves and muscles to ensure they're firing on all cylinders and conveying accurate messages. If you don't do this then you can't expect your pelvic floor Kegels to have their best effect or work for you as well as they did for your friend, sister or mum. This is called neuromuscular control or simply 'muscle memory', where you restore your nerve-to-muscle connections, find all your pelvic floor muscles and feel the action of each one. Instead of assuming we all know how to do our pelvic floor exercises, let's assume we don't and are setting up messages from our brain to these precious parts for the very first time.

Often you're told to perform your pelvic floor exercise throughout the day, while you're sat in traffic, feeding your baby or working at your desk, but the truth is that will only maintain the strength you already have and is unlikely to progress you further. Muscle building is more intense than this, especially following the strain of pregnancy and birth, and at first it's unlikely you'll be able to breathe at the same time, let alone nurse a baby or drive a car!

In pregnancy the weight of our full uterus on our pelvic floor, the swelling in our legs and groin, and perhaps any varicose veins that appeared are all physical signs of compromised blood flow down there. Where the blood cannot flow freely, neither can the nerve impulses, so our pelvic floor contractions need practising more frequently to keep them strong. Sadly, we can't assume they're doing what they have always done when our bodies are so different now. Exercising through pregnancy is one way of ensuring the nerve-to-muscle connections stay strong despite skeletal changes, but don't worry, exercising after birth is another.

During birth, whether you have an abdominal or vaginal delivery, there will be some degree of nerve trauma. This can range from being temporarily stunned when your baby passes through the birth canal to longer lasting numbness and dysfunction as a result of surgery or manual intervention. When the nerves are stretched, cut or moved, their firing capacity can be dulled, delayed or impaired. This can last just a few seconds, much like waking up with a dead arm that you've been sleeping on, or it can last several hours, days or even weeks. You may have little to no sensation and/or little to no power. I have met many mums who, after giving birth, experienced zero control of their bladders every time they stood up or – the other extreme – unable to pass urine and dependent on catheters to relieve themselves for weeks, even after they were discharged home. This may happen when the baby's head has been sitting in the birth canal for an extended period of time in a slow second stage, so instead of just a few seconds, many minutes may go by with the nerves compressed, stretched and distorted. It can take a while for the nerve-to-muscle to work again due to this temporary nerve palsy. The extent of this and its duration will give some indication of the recovery and rehabilitation the nerve and muscle connection needs.

Inflammation is another important feature affecting our neuromuscular control following birth, an injury or an operation. Inflammation is the first stage in any healing process. When we cut, tear or over stretch any part of our body, fluid known as 'lymph' is sent to the area to initiate healing. Lymph is our body's healing soup, filled with immune cells, hormones and nutrients to fix the problem, but once flooded with this soup our nerve and muscle connection becomes dull. The signalling cannot get through and, as a result, feeling and control of the injured muscles can be lost. This is completely normal and our body's way of protecting us from further injury. As our body heals, the inflammation gradually subsides and so should last no more than 2–3 weeks. If loss of function and feeling goes beyond this time, it is likely there are other features involved that we need to consider in order to heal and rebuild.

And so strengthening begins with practising our brain-nerve-muscle connection to ensure that what we *think* we are doing is actually happening. The aim is to recruit every muscle layer, from superficial to deep, left to right, back passage to the front passage, and then to fully let go, release and relax.

TASK 4 PELVIC FLOOR EXERCISES FOR LIFE

KIT YOU WILL NEED: Some time to yourself and somewhere comfortable to sit or lie where you feel relaxed and safe.

Start trying this while you're lying on your back with your knees bent and ensure your tail is not tucked under. When you can, progress this into sitting, kneeling and then eventually to standing. If you always do your pelvic floor exercises lying down, then these muscles will be super-strong here, but not up against gravity where you need them the most. (Remember to wash your hands just in case you find that you need to feel your way around).

Finding your pelvic floor muscles – all three layers, from the front to the back, left to right, both up and down – can feel tough to begin with. Start with the position in which you can feel your pelvic floor responding most easily. Try sitting on a gym ball, where you have the pressure and feedback from the ball's surface against your external pelvic floor, or lying down, where there is no weight pressing down on the hammock. Lying on your tummy is another good position to try this in as it tips your sacrum, therefore pelvis and consequently your pelvic floor, into a locked position, but be cautious if you have an abdominal scar from a Caesarean birth and don't do this if it's painful.

Isolate your back passage. Imagine, touch or look at your anus in a mirror. What you can see on the outside is the external muscles only. Behind this lie even more layers of pelvic floor muscle, lifting and kinking the rectum and pulling your tail towards your pubic bone. Let's start to find and use these muscles layer by layer. Starting at the outside layer, squeeze these muscles like you would your lips when sucking up spaghetti. Tighten this outside muscle like pursing your lips. Hold and add in the next layer of muscle by imagining sucking that spaghetti a little inside. Finally, engage the deepest part of the back passage and pelvic floor by sucking that spaghetti all the way up. Don't try and hold, just try to get there. Now release your contraction from the deep layer, then middle layer and finally the outside layer. Don't push the spaghetti out, just let it go so that it falls back down on to your plate!

Next do the same for your vaginal canal. Imagine, touch or look at the outside. This is your vulva, but if you part the labia you can see the start of your vaginal canal. Your vagina extends from here all the way up to the neck of your womb and is flanked by the pelvic floor muscles. Imagine how a jelly fish swims. It tightens the muscles of its body to push itself upwards, contracting its muscular body from the bottom/outside, upwards, pushing itself higher. Try to tighten the pelvic floor muscles around the vaginal canal in the same way. Do this layer by layer, from the outside or opening of the vagina, then adding in the middle layer, tightening the vaginal canal and finally the deepest layer as though you are pinching the neck of the womb. Don't hold it. Just get it there. Then release it downwards, layer by layer, like the jellyfish, moving back down through the water gradually, without falling, until you can finally release all the muscles.

Finally try this with your urethra (the tube which carries urine away from the bladder). The opening sits just behind the pubic bone under the top fold of your labia, before your vaginal opening. Again, it's a good idea to touch here or take a look to establish a good conscious awareness of this part of the pelvic floor muscle. Imagine a zipper, like that on a pair of jeans, running from here, up the inside of your tummy, to your belly button. Use your muscles to pinch the outside opening of the urethra, as though you're taking hold of the zip. Then 'zip up' the whole front wall of the pelvic floor, pulling this zipper upwards, tightening bit by bit up the length of your urethra until you can feel yourself lifting your bladder upwards. Then unzip gradually, with as much conscious control as you used to zip up. Finally, let go of the pinch of the outside muscles and release the zip from your grasp.

Try just a few of each to start with and build up to at least 10 on each passageway. It will likely feel hard to access every muscle layer at the start, but remember that you are retraining what you have struggled to do, so it should feel difficult at the beginning and will take concentration. Repeat 2-3 times every day until it feels easy.

Women sometimes tell me that their front or deep pelvic floor contraction feels weaker than the back or outside and sometimes it's the reverse. Either way, our goal is to build up all three layers, front, middle and back, from the outside to the deepest layer, so that each feels just as strong as the other. We need to ensure that we are working the whole muscle before we move onwards. Repeat this frequently and you will soon start to get feedback from the muscle that it is doing as you ask.

Once you can find and feel all of your pelvic floor working we can start to consider the muscle as a whole and work it to achieve our maximum strength and endurance. For true muscle strengthening we need to recruit every muscle fibre or layer we have, hold each contraction for as long as we can and complete as many repetitions as possible before we feel tired. The goal is to work all passageways together, not just one at a time.

Let's try the 'vaginal elevator' I mentioned at the start of this book. Trying it again now you know so much more about your body can make it feel like a whole new exercise!

The three-stage lift:

1.   Imagine the pelvic floor as an elevator with doors at the pelvic outlet. When the doors are open the pelvic floor muscles are relaxed. Tighten the superficial

muscles, those at your body's outlets, to close the doors, sliding the muscles together from right to left or left to right. Once you feel the 'doors' are firmly closed you can start to pull the elevator up into your pelvis.

2.   Lift the elevator to the first floor and pause here, feeling the middle layer of your pelvic floor hammock tighten and lift up inside your body. Keep the doors shut.

3.   Then, keeping the doors closed, lift the elevator even higher up to engage the deepest of your pelvic floor muscles. You should feel your pelvic organs being lifted up to your top floor by your 'vaginal elevator'.

The three-stage lower:

1.   Once you've reached your highest lift, lower the elevator down to the first floor, slowly and steadily.

2.   Now lower the elevator even further, keeping just the doors closed and your pelvic outlets pinched.

3.   When you have relaxed from the inside out you can finally open the doors and allow the contraction to release fully and let go. Often we can forget to 'open the doors' and hold on to a little contraction because of anxiety, pain or even eagerness to 'perform'. To fully open the doors, try breathing out and saying 'Ahhhh,' relaxing your jaw to let the muscle go.

I often demonstrate this contraction with my hands and you can try it yourself. Take the index finger of your left hand and wrap your right hand around it, palm facing towards you. Imagine your right hand is your pelvic floor muscle that runs around your vaginal wall and your left finger is examining what the muscle is doing. Squeeze your left finger with the muscles on the outside of your imaginary vagina, tightening your right hand around your left, starting with the little finger. Continue to wrap the right hand around the left finger one by one, imaginary pelvic floor muscle layer by imaginary pelvic floor muscle layer, until you are squeezing right up to the tip of your finger. This is exactly what I can feel when I assess pelvic floor strength internally. This may help you to transfer the same segmental lifting action to the pelvic floor. Give it a try!

STEP 3

Once you've got the hang of the three-stage lift and three-stage lower it's time to build endurance, so you need to hold your best contraction for as long as you can. The 'gold standard' and recommendation from the National Institute for Clinical

Excellence (NICE) is to hold for 10 seconds x10. However, my advice is not to stop at 10 seconds if that feels easy, nor even just 10 repetitions, but to hold and repeat until you start to tire. This is known as fatigue. True strength comes from fatiguing the muscle we already have, stimulating our body to respond and build more muscle.

What does fatigue of your pelvic floor muscles feel like? When your contractions are not as strong as they were when you started, when you find it harder to recruit or release all of the muscle, or when your endurance starts to fade on each repetition you have reached fatigue. This may happen after two repetitions of 10 seconds or 20 repetitions of six seconds. The point is it's personal to you. Note that this may be different each day too. If you've been more active or have had little sleep you may become fatigued more quickly than you do on another day. This is totally OK! As long as you fully relax after each contraction, every effort will be a step towards your goal. If you perform your contractions in this way – to fatigue – then you need to do this just once every day, much like going to the gym. Doing it thoroughly and once a day is plenty when you aim for muscle fatigue rather than a number.

Is my tummy working too much?

We are often told that our tummy muscles shouldn't work at all when we perform pelvic floor contractions and we should be able to do them anywhere, anytime, without anyone else noticing. While this is true for a sub-maximal contraction, one that keeps the strength you already have, this type of contraction will not grow a bigger muscle and therefore won't provide any greater strength than you have already. What you are practising here is a maximal contraction, which goes beyond what you find easy to recruit and develops all the muscles, from the outside of your pelvic floor to the deepest layer, from the very back to the very front. When you do this you should also feel your lower tummy pull in, sometimes all the way up to your belly button. Your tummy should never bulge outwards or downwards with this contraction, but just slightly lift and pull a tiny bit flatter. The most important thing to watch for is that you feel your pelvic floor muscles first, so stages 1 and 2 are all on the inside, and your lower tummy pulls up and in only when you engage stage 3, the deepest layer, and not before.

When or how do I breathe?

This is the next question I am asked when I teach pelvic floor exercises or I often hear the statement, 'I can't breathe and do this.' Of course you can't – or not at first anyway. You are re-training a nerve-to-muscle connection and only when you have established this can you incorporate your breath. When you're ready here's how to incorporate your breathing and, most importantly, your diaphragmatic lift.

Breathe in and notice the pelvic floor's relaxed starting point. Then, as you begin to breathe out, start your pelvic floor contraction and keep breathing out as you lift up layer by layer, through stages 1, 2 and 3. As you breathe out the diaphragm moves up and so does the pelvic floor. Pause at the top of your contraction and try to breathe in and out gently, while maintaining your best pelvic floor contraction. Then slowly breathe out again as you lower your contraction back down to rest, through stages 3, 2 and then 1. If this is too fast, or you need more breath, that's OK. Breathe when you need to. Try not to take in your fullest breaths, which is a challenge in itself, but just your normal breathing pattern, so you are training your pelvic floor under 'normal' circumstances.

Within four weeks of performing task 4 daily you should feel the nerve-to-muscle connection again. During these exercises you should sense the tightening of the pelvic floor and when you relax you should feel you can do so fully, layer by layer, within just a few seconds. If this isn't happening after the first four to six weeks, if you continue not to feel your pelvic floor contractions, and if your body doesn't tell you to go to the bathroom and you find your underwear is wet or soiled, then it is likely that the nerves will need further assistance to heal. At this point I would urge you to visit your doctor or a women's health physiotherapist in person. Following their assessment, they may recommend further help in the shape of various gadgets and gizmos to help your nerves and muscle connect, heal and rebuild.

Pelvic floor gadgets and gizmos

Fear not, these tools are not essential to your healing and rebuilding. They are only there if you fancy trying them out or feel you need some extra help, but we can train your pelvic floor without them.

Muscle stimulation

Do you remember those tummy tighteners of the 1990s? The ones which promised washboard abs? They were belts around your waist with electrical stimulation pads. They would send signals to the muscles, bypassing the nerves and making the abdominals contract. We can do the same thing for the pelvic floor through a clinical device known as neuro muscular electrical stimulation (NMES). Kegel 8, Neurotrac and Pericalm are all products designed to improve your pelvic floor's neuromuscular connection and ultimately resting tone and strength. Through tampon-like probes inserted into the vagina, electrical impulses are transmitted from the gadget's hand-held device directly to the pelvic floor muscle. Instead of the brain and its peripheral nerves conveying messages to contract, these magical devices do all the firing up instead, getting straight to the problematic area.

NMES is recommended when pelvic floor strength is grade 2 or below on the scale, so when there is an inconsistent pelvic floor muscle contraction, just a flicker or no palpable contraction. At grade 2 you are unlikely to be able to enroll enough of your muscles with the contraction you have to make it stronger. You need to involve a greater number of muscle fibres to get a bigger and more effective contraction. NMES is an essential way of maximising muscle recruitment and getting you to a grade 3 on the strength scale, where you can do your exercises on your own. I recommend using NMES while performing Task 4 daily for 6 to 12 weeks, after which you are likely to be ready to exercise without NMES.

If you have recently had a baby or gynaecological surgery, in order to prevent infection you shouldn't use insertable devices until your wounds are fully healed. However, Kegel 8 and a product called Innovo offer external stimulation options, meaning they deliver NMES via electrodes placed on your skin, bypassing the vagina and going straight to the source – the sacral nerves in your back and bottom which supply your bladder, bowel and pelvic floor muscles. Sacral nerve stimulation sends signals along these nerves to the muscle directly making them contract, even in the presence of injury. If you need to, or when you feel ready, you can also combine this approach with internal probes once your internal scars have healed. You'll then be bombarding the nerve and muscle pathway both up the chain directly from the muscle and down the chain via the nerve, thereby maximising the healing and rebuilding.

Biofeedback

If you are new to these contractions, still have reduced sensation or would just like to make sure your time spent exercising these muscles is efficient, you may like to use a biofeedback tool. Pelvic floor biofeedback is a technique that lets you know exactly what's going on down there when you squeeze and lift. These insertable tools send visual or sensory information in response to your pelvic floor muscle action. When you contract, they move, light up, vibrate, sing or dance. Some are like computer games for your vagina – you tighten in response to what you see on your phone or computer screen to meet targets and goals. My favourite is the one I experienced at my first NHS women's health check-up. My vagina was linked up to a computer screen and my pelvic floor came to life as a bee, cruising around a field of flowers. All the flower heads were at different heights and as I contracted my pelvic floor the bee moved upwards. I completed a series of tasks, contracting and releasing my pelvic floor just enough to visit as many flower heads as I could, which made it all a bit more fun. Not only was this enjoyable, but I was also seeing for the first time what my pelvic floor could do – and it was a lot more than I was giving it credit for! This extra reassurance and feedback may be just what you need to keep you motivated and on track.

There are many of these biofeedback tools on the market. While they won't do your exercises for you or provide any sort of resistance, they are designed to give you a greater sense of what is happening when you do your 'pelvic floors'. The Elvie trainer, Neen pelvic floor educator, Vibrance pelvic trainer and Perifit are all portable tools you can buy and use at home. They will provide you with feedback, acting like your own portable women's health physiotherapist. You can use them every time you do your exercises to give you instant feedback on the accuracy and strength of your contraction, or just every now and again to check you're improving. The instant feedback you get is both encouraging and motivating.

Cones, weights and toners

Once the nerve-to-muscle connection has been re-established, we can add resistance, repetition and task-specific training. OK, so now you have a good three-stage contraction that you can hold for at least 10 seconds x10. Is this enough to grow a bigger muscle and resolve overstretch or injury? For some yes, completely, but others will need to work harder. How strong you need your pelvic floor to be depends on what you're asking it to do. If you're feeling stronger yet still experiencing symptoms when you have a cough, exercise or have a rare night out, then you're not yet 'strong enough'. Adding some resistance to your three-stage contraction and 'pelvic floor exercises for life' will push your strength further. To have more strength you need more muscle fibres all pulling in the same direction; not bulging bicep-like vaginal muscles, but firm, dense muscles. We apply this principle to every muscle in the body during rehabilitation and the pelvic floor is no different.

So the next step in pelvic floor strengthening is to add weights or resistance – what physiotherapists call 'load'. Unlike other muscles in the body, the pelvic floor cannot lift weights or kettle bells. I rarely recommend using weighted eggs or cones as these can unhelpfully build overactivity and high tone in the muscles, which won't allow the essential relaxation phase to happen. We want the resistance to be there when contracting, but we also want to release fully between repetitions. This is hard to do when you've inserted a heavy weight into the vagina and you don't want it to drop out when you relax! We need a tool that can close or change shape in response to our squeeze, resist our squeeze so that we need to put in more effort and then stay in place as we relax ready for the next exercise. For this I regularly recommend the Pelvic Toner. It's a spring-loaded device that looks a bit like curling tongs. You press it closed to insert it into your vagina. Once inside it opens and takes up the vaginal space. As you perform your exercises in task 4, you will gradually close and tighten your muscles against the spring's resistance. You can even use your hands on the hinge of the handle to check the toner is closing. Work on holding it there, without it opening up, keeping your contraction and closure on the toner steady, and then release it fully, allowing it to open, before repeating. While you're aiming for 10 seconds x10, you can stop when you get tired, when you can't hold for the full 10 seconds, you can't close it as fully as you were doing or you can't sense your contraction as you did previously. Here's the best part, though: when you can achieve this you can increase the load further, just like going for a heavier weight in the gym. There's a range of resistance springs and you can add more than one to challenge the pelvic floor as you progress.

One day I plan to create a device that can give resistance like the toner, feedback like a women's health physiotherapist, electrical stimulation when its needed and still be discreet, motivating and fun! Until then you may need more than one device to support you on your healing and rebuilding journey.

If the idea of pelvic floor paraphernalia doesn't feel right for you, that's totally fine – it's just one way of helping you work the muscles so that they are fit for function. There is another way to approach this and that's through adding an external load or weight. Pilates circles, balls, adductor machines – all of these will fire up your inside thigh. Like the pelvic floor, your inner thighs attach to the pubic bone and help with pelvic floor, pelvic ring and tummy closure. Likewise, when you add a resistance band around the outside of the legs and press outwards, you fire up your hip external rotators, which close and stabilise the back of your pelvis, the sacro-iliac joints and ultimately your posterior pelvic floor. Working with these tools *alongside* your pelvic floor exercises will maximise the loading of your pelvic floor to tighten and grow more muscles where you need them.

True pelvic floor strength requires us to consider strength throughout our body – what we call 'global' strength. So when I said the pelvic floor cannot lift weights and kettle bells, that's not strictly true. The floor of the pelvis is involved in every movement we make. When we squat our pelvic floor muscles are working; if we do a kettle bell swing, so does our pelvic floor; if we power out on the cross trainer for 20 minutes so do our pelvic floor muscles. This means we need to train our pelvic floor in proportion to life's challenges.

TASK 5 KETTLE BELL KEGELS

KIT YOU WILL NEED: Weights, a bag of books, a toddler or just gravity.

We've started all our tasks so far lying down, where they're easiest, where the pelvic floor doesn't need to support the pelvic organs and gravity is our friend, but this is not a functional training position. I'm sure you don't get your worst symptoms when you're lying down. We need to build up to the most challenging positions, adding gravity and external weights as resistance. In all the following scenarios, perform your pelvic floor exercises as previously, in three stages.

Your goal is to hold the effort for 10 seconds x10. When you have achieved this, move on to the next exercise. Stop progressing when things feel too hard and add on the next levels only when you feel you can. It's not about how far you get, but how good you get at each exercise.

Prone heel squeeze: Lying on your tummy naturally tips your pelvis forwards, thereby creating tension in your pelvic floor just by lying there. In this position rest your forehead on your hands and do your pelvic floor exercises while pressing your heels firmly together. Your bottom, lower back, tummy and inner thigh muscles will kick in and work with your pelvic floor.

Four-point heel squeeze: On your hands and knees, try not to tuck your tail under but release your tail out, so that the natural curves in your back are present but not exaggerated. Now perform your pelvic floor exercises, firmly squeezing your heels together as you go. All of your deep hip stabilisers are working, as well as your pelvic floor. When you can hold the effort for 10 seconds x10, add a ball between your knees and squeeze this at the same time to recruit your inner thigh muscles too.

Perched squat: Start perched on the edge of a chair, bench or table with your tail out and ball between your knees. Lean slightly forwards, as though you are about to stand up. Squeeze the ball and press down through your feet as you complete your pelvic floor exercises. As soon as you can, start to hover your bottom just one inch off of the chair and isolate your pelvic floor muscles here.

Weighted: When you can handle the three positions above it's time to add more load in the form of free weights. Start with just 2-4kg in total (about the weight of a newborn baby!). Perform movements that are close to the body and don't require you to move at your hips, such as bicep curls or lateral raises. Hold the same standing posture and each time you lift the weight squeeze, close and lift your pelvic floor. Try squeezing the ball between your knees at the same time for even greater muscle recruitment.

Squats: So we've added multiple muscles, gravity and weights. Now we add movement. We need strength not just when we are in one position, but in many positions. When we squat, we bend our hips and knees, tip our pelvis, engage the muscles in our back, thighs and tummy, and mobilise our pelvic floor. What we achieve is perfect multi-tasking for high level pelvic floor training. Hold a ball between your knees, and maybe even add some free weights in your hands (a few bags of flour or sugar in a backpack works if you don't have fancy weights). Bend your knees and hips, reaching your arms forwards. Try to keep your knees in line with your ankles and not collapse them forwards. Before you stand back up, squeeze the ball, engage the pelvic floor and breathe out as you stand. Release, repeat. Before you progress, aim for at least x20 without tiring.

Move through these steps as you grow stronger. It's not the passing of time that builds the strength, but the adaptations our bodies make to build strength as we go. Don't be tempted to skip stages!

Your tailor-made pelvic floor programme is a combination of what you find most challenging. If you're finding the exercises easy, but you're still having symptoms, then you're not working at the right level and it's time to move on. Your body will respond to this training, just like preparing for a race. You don't start off running your longest distance. Instead you break down what you need to be able to do and work up to it. I promise you can get there by keeping at it and progressing a little at a time as you find the exercises becoming too easy.

Real-life story

Ava is a mum of two on earth, two in heaven, and a runner

The birth of our son couldn't have been more straightforward, which came as a huge surprise after the challenges we had to get there. Following the loss of our twins at 20 weeks' gestation I struggled to fall pregnant again. When I did, it was a pregnancy filled with anxiety. I was thrilled to have a baby boy and his birth was easy in comparison to the challenges I had overcome. I had a small tear, which was easily stitched, and everything seemed fine. My six-week check with the GP came and went, with more questions about contraception than my physical health. I was too embarrassed to mention the constant feeling of needing to go to the loo and the frequent wet patch in my underwear. I figured both would sort themselves out in time and kept up with my pelvic floor exercises, which in hindsight I wish someone had taught me at the beginning, as I know now I wasn't doing them right.

So three months after giving birth and with my knickers no drier, I was shocked to suddenly feel like my insides were falling out and I could feel something protruding from my vagina. I was worried and upset when my GP diagnosed pelvic floor weakness and a prolapse. Despite the endless ante-natal appointments (many more than normal because of my previous late miscarriage) and an NCT course, this was the first time I'd ever heard about a prolapse. I had no idea what I was dealing with. My GP said I should just continue with the pelvic floor exercises I had been doing and gave me something to help with the constipation that had plagued my pregnancy and was still bothering me – something I also thought I just had to put up with and hadn't mentioned to anyone. I had no idea that this was hampering my pelvic floor recovery.

My biggest fear was that I would no longer be able to run. I'm not an elite athlete by any stretch of the imagination, but running has been my main way of destressing and keeping myself sane for many years. Before trying for a family, I ran half marathons and a long run of 10 or more miles was always part of my weekend. I was scared of the idea that I would never be able to run again because of my pelvic floor.

It made sense to me to start with physiotherapy when my BuggyFit trainer recommended this. From my first appointment my pelvic floor and I had a clear plan to recover and run again. Over the next six months I put my body through its paces to build the strength in my pelvic floor and core for the life I wanted to lead. I invested in a pelvic toner, which is a brilliant gadget for telling me I am doing everything correctly. Like in any other training regime, the exercises got harder with time, I could feel my strength improving, and with this I was feeling relieved and reassured. I tentatively started running again. I was careful to build up slowly and not push myself too hard; to work within what my body could do and what I had trained it for.

Just after our son turned one, I was amazed to find that I was pregnant again. After all the difficulties of the past, our daughter arrived after an uneventful pregnancy and a birth almost as quick as her brother's. I confess that, despite knowing full well that I should do pelvic floor exercises while I was pregnant, I rarely found the time. With a one year old and a busy full-time job, I neglected them. But once our daughter arrived, I knew I needed to rebuild my strength for the long term, even if there were no immediate problems.

I started doing my exercises again, but my rebuilding plan was tougher to stick to the second time around. I was tired and suffered with back pain as a result of my weakened core, but I stuck with it and slowly started to feel myself get stronger. The journey back to running started after six months – three months sooner than first time around. My physio taught me to support my pelvic floor with pessaries while running. Like wearing a support on any other body part, I used these internally to protect me from injury and I continued to work on building my strength to cope without them. Before long I didn't need the pessaries anymore and I returned to running with dry knickers. I feel strong now and although I don't run as far or quite as fast as I did before my children, running continues to be a big part of my life. If I have learnt anything over the last four years, it's that physical strength is worth far more than physical appearance.

When to ask for help:

- You don't feel right downstairs, and your body doesn't feel or act in a way that is right for you.
- You leak urine, wind or poo, whether it's only a few days or a few years after birth. There isn't a time frame – this is a sign of injury, big or small.
- You feel there is something in your vagina, it feels like something is falling out or your insides feel heavy. You may have a pelvic organ prolapse and you need support to manage this.
- You suspect that your pelvic floor muscles may be too tense and are struggling to relax despite the tasks in this book.

What to ask for:

- Start here. The advice in this book may be enough for you to heal and rebuild. If you need more support I encourage you to begin with women's health physiotherapy as the first treatment for all these problems. If you need investigation or further help we can point you in the right direction.

What's important

- Restoring pelvic floor function is a step by step process. Pelvic floor training should follow the same process as for any other part of the body.
- A strong pelvic floor is one that can both contract and relax fully. We need to be able to move the muscles through a full range, all the way up and all the way down, in order for them to keep up with the rest of our body.

Release: Let it go

- It's essential that we establish what a relaxed pelvic floor feels like before we start 'tightening it'.
- It's a little-known fact that just as many pelvic floor symptoms arise from pelvic floors that are too tense as those which are too lax.
- Stretches and exercise can be effective enough in restoring normal resting tone, providing a good baseline from which to rebuild.

Strengthening: Find it, feel it, contract, hold, release, repeat

- Practise various ways to find and work the front, middle and back of the pelvic floor in all its three stages.
- Repeat the exercises in various positions, particularly those you find most difficult.
- Once you've found and restored a good through-range contraction, hold it to build endurance.
- Repeat, repeat, repeat. Don't stop when you hit a number, but when you start to tire. Only then will your muscles change. It's unlikely you will feel that familiar post-workout muscle ache in your pelvic floor as it is a slow twitch muscle. Instead you know you have worked your muscle to fatigue when:
  - Your contraction doesn't feel as strong as the one before.
  - You can't hold the contraction as long as the one before.
  - You can no longer feel a clear release and relax between your pelvic floor contractions.
  - You start to use other muscles to achieve the same connection (bottom-gripping or thigh-tensing are the most common!).

Muscle-building: Load it

- Adding some weight or 'load' will further strengthen your pelvic floor to match the resistance of life's challenges (carrying a toddler springs to mind!).

- A more powerful muscle means a bigger muscle and the only way to grow a bigger muscle is by adding a load; some sort of resistance in order to tire the body and encourage new muscle growth.

- Training in this way is a daily process and it will take a minimum of three months to see and feel the difference.

Tools to aid pelvic floor rehabilitation

Biofeedback

- When: 'Am I doing it right?' or 'I'm doing it right, but I just can't hold it.'
- Tools: Neen pelvic floor educator, Elvie Trainer, Perifit, Joy ON.

Neuromuscular Electrical Stimulation (NMES)

- When: 'I can't feel it' or 'My physiotherapist says I'm very weak.'
- Tools: Kegel 8, Innovo, Neutotrac.

Resistance

- When: 'I'm doing it right, but I'm still getting symptoms' or 'I'm fine unless…'
- Tools: Pelvic Toner.

4. Birth injuries: Those that you can't put a plaster on

With nine out of 10 vaginal births in first-time mothers resulting in cuts or tears to the nether regions, it is not just newborn babies who need tender loving care following their arrival. For many of us this will be our first encounter with pain and injury. And while navigating a path we never expected to take seems scary, we must trust that our body will heal. Birth injuries such as episiotomies, perineal tears, forceps-related birth canal trauma and vaginal muscle injuries are often swept under the carpet as being part and parcel of childbirth.

As a physiotherapist I can assure you that injuries to the body's other muscles, tendons and joints are never treated with such disdain. We need to start treating the physical traumas of childbirth as we would injuries to any other part of the body. If you get a cut or a graze anywhere else, I bet that not a day goes by without you inspecting it. If you strain or tear a muscle I am sure you would be guided by your pain on when to return to activity, and with serious injury you would seek professional advice before jumping straight back into your chosen sport. Yet too often I hear that women are too scared or too worried to properly examine their birth wounds. They cannot recall being told about the severity of their injuries or how to care for them. It is hard to navigate our physical recovery if we are unaware of exactly what our bodies have been through. How can we nurture, heal and restore if we are unsure about what we're dealing with?

No matter how long ago our birth(s), it is likely that signs of our labour(s) remain. Once we are familiar with these we can work on nurturing, repairing and restoring strength where it's needed. Take a look at the rest of your body – are there scars or marks from injuries sustained as a child or previous surgeries? These scars fade, our bodies heal, but it's likely those physical reminders remain visible. If you haven't before then I urge you to grab a mirror and travel south. While this might feel silly, or even scary, you will see that birth injuries often feel much worse than they are. If you have recently given birth, taking a look down there will help you to keep the wound clean, monitor your healing progress and support you with your pelvic floor exercises. If some time has passed since your child's birth then it may surprise you that you can still see signs of assisted deliveries, cuts or tears. Although they have healed, there may be scar tissue left behind and, if you can still see scars, perhaps you can still feel them too.

So what are you looking for and where is it?

Episiotomies

These are surgical incisions or cuts from the vaginal opening out towards the buttock muscle, made to give our baby's head more space to birth and to avoid a spontaneous tear which could damage our anal canal. They are performed by an obstetric doctor with surgical scissors and you are given lots of pain relief. If you haven't had an epidural at this point then local anaesthetic will be injected into and around your perineum. With a 'posterior-lateral' incision – meaning to the back and side, often the right side as most surgeons are right-handed – an episiotomy preserves the precious perineum, the security guard of your anus. With the perineum intact our anus and it's precious sphincter muscle, which we only have one, remains whole and protected from injury. However, there may instead be some trauma to the pelvic floor muscles of which we have many and while this is considered the lesser of two evils, the recovery from an episiotomy is akin to that of a second degree tear.

You will find your episiotomy scar either at 5 or 7 o'clock if you imagine the opening of the birth canal as a clock face. It gives the vaginal opening a lopsided, down turned smile - which is quite appropriate given the injury. Depending on how long ago you gave birth this will look anything from a prominent, red, raised ridge to a thin, faint, white line.

While an episiotomy isn't guaranteed to protect you from a perineal tear, it does make one less likely. However, it isn't always possible or appropriate to perform an episiotomy if your baby's head is delivered too hard and fast or if you have your baby at home without a doctor or midwife present to intervene.

External Female Genitalia

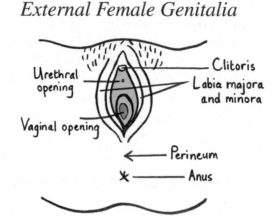

Urethral opening

Clitoris

Labia majora and minora

Vaginal opening

Perineum

Anus

Birth Injuries

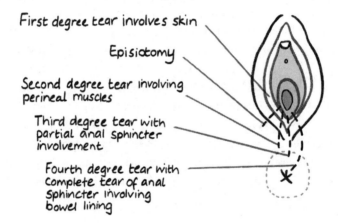

First degree tear involves skin

Episiotomy

Second degree tear involving perineal muscles

Third degree tear with partial anal sphincter involvement

Fourth degree tear with complete tear of anal sphincter involving bowel lining

Perineal tears

A perineal tear tends to extend directly back from the vaginal opening towards the bottom, straight through the perineal body. Though tears and grazes (those which just affect the skin) can extend outwards from any part of the vaginal opening, those that extend straight back is the most common. There are many risk factors for perineal tearing; from the size of your baby to the speed of your labour; the amount of pain relief you have to the position you birth in. You may feel as though your baby has bashed his or her way into this world, storming past the perineal guard and leaving your back passage vulnerable. In hindsight you may wish you had done things differently, but the truth is it's difficult if not impossible to predict who will sustain a birth injury in labour and who will not. Here's the important part: our bodies are amazing and you will heal. There's also plenty we can do to enhance your recovery, so that in time you will feel stronger than ever.

Perineal tears are graded according to their depth and what structures are involved:

First degree: Involving just the skin, these can be called 'grazes' and while they are sore and sting, they tend to heal quickly and do not require repair.

Second degree: These involve the skin and muscle underneath, and they do need stitching and pelvic floor muscle rehabilitation. The repair is often performed in the same delivery room that you gave birth in. It's worth noting that episiotomies may also involve some of the pelvic floor muscle and their healing should be considered comparable to that of a second degree tear.

Third degree: These involve injury to the skin, muscle and the anal sphincter. A grade 3a tear involves less than 50% of the external anal sphincter, 3b involves more than 50% and a 3c is where both the external and internal anal sphincter (IAS) are torn. These will be repaired in theatre by an obstetric or gynaecological doctor. For a third degree tear, pelvic floor rehabilitation with a physiotherapist is essential and a follow-up with a specialist 'perineal trauma clinic' should be arranged for you before you leave hospital.

Fourth degree: This is a tear of the skin, muscle, both the internal and external anal sphincters, and into the anal canal itself. Like a third degree tear, fourth degree tears are referred to as obstetric anal sphincter injuries (OASIS). Unlike the serenity normally associated with an oasis, this type of tear can quickly turn your birth haven into a medical drama. They require immediate and precise surgery to repair both the back passage and vaginal wall to prevent poo passing into your vagina. You will be given significant follow-up care to ensure complete recovery of your vagina, your anal sphincter and its canal, and to restore your pelvic floor muscles.

Protect

Regardless of the type of birth trauma, whether you have sustained an injury at all or if you feel your birth trauma is emotional rather than physical, post-birth recovery takes time. Every birth and delivery is unique, challenging and preceded by a pregnancy from which you need to heal.

The first few weeks after delivery are an important time in everyone's healing. Our bodies have altered greatly during this last year, and the new and sudden changes can be a shock. Pain and inflammation make us move and function differently to normal. We need to give ourselves time to heal, to protect our posture and to restore our strength.

Take this opportunity to rest at home. While it may be tempting, don't rush out for a walk or race to get either you or your baby dressed. Remember you are healing an injury like anywhere else in the body. Pain and discomfort are messages from your body telling you to take things easy. Listen to them. Even at home, limit the time you spend on your feet. Fighting against gravity can make things feel heavier and more swollen down there. Instead, try perching on the bath to brush your teeth, fold the laundry from the edge of your bed, prepare food, bottles and toddler snacks while sitting down. Better still call on your family and friends to help with whatever they can. I'm sure they'd love to.

When you are ready to get dressed, keep your clothes loose and as natural as possible. You want to avoid any seams that will create pressure or friction against the perineum. Also avoid anything too tight or too warm. This can increase the risk of swelling and infection.

Set yourself up with all the comforts, equipment and supplies you need for you and your baby, on one floor if possible, so that you don't even have to tackle stairs. This will minimise the movement through the pelvis and pelvic floor. Allow your baby to be brought to you and try not to walk around the house carrying him or her. Beautiful as they are, they're a heavy weight on your healing parts.

With your time now taken up with a demanding little one, finding time and even remembering to support our own healing can be a challenge. Here's a quick checklist for *everyone* to enhance recovery during those first few weeks post-birth:

- Accept all the help offered. Your body needs to heal and you need to get to know your baby. Perhaps your birth didn't go quite as expected and it will take time to process the dramatic events. Feel supported so that you can prioritise yourself and your baby.

- Drink like a fish. Our bodies are 60% water so we need to ensure that we have plenty for new tissue growth and healing. If you are breast feeding you also need to take on more water for making breast milk too. Every time your baby takes a feed from you, replenish with a glass of water for yourself.

- Avoid constipation. Even though you may not want to think about it, pooing (or more accurately not pooing) is very impactful on our recovery after pregnancy and birth. A heavy, full bowel will put the pelvic hammock under strain, stretching the healing tissues and giving the compromised pelvic floor muscles extra weight to carry around. Hard stools are difficult to pass and can lead to anal trauma, straining, haemorrhoids and prolapse. In summary, constipation is the arch-nemesis of perineal healing and why your midwife keeps asking about your bowel movements! If you haven't already been given them, ask your doctor for laxatives or a stool softener. Continue taking these for at least the first 2–3 week acute healing phase so that poo can pass more easily and take some strain off your healing perineum. A squatty potty or child's stool to rest your feet on is also a good option in the early days. This puts a gentle stretch on your pelvic floor and helps your poo to drop down more easily.

- Apply cold compresses three times a day for the first 2–3 weeks. Freezing your maternity pads is a super-simple way of doing this. Cooling the area helps with blood flow to your injury. That knee jerk withdrawal as you feel the cold on your skin is exactly what your blood vessels need to do. They constrict and withdraw, and as they warm up they dilate again. This pumping action brings all the nutrients to the area and carries whatever is not supporting healing away.

- Offload your perineum as much as you can and try not to sit directly on your swollen bits. Weight on any scars and healing tissues will not only feel sore, but will reduce the blood flow where it is needed the most. Lying on your side to feed (bottle or breast) is not only easiest for you and your baby, but also helps the blood and all its healing nutrients to get down there. Lying on your back with your legs elevated or lying on your tummy are also great positions for you. When you have to sit, make what my friend Hayley called the gutter pillow! It's as simple as rolling two towels and placing one under each buttock, keeping weight off the perineum. You can use horse-shoe shaped feeding pillows for this too or even a rubber ring.

- Keep out of your pre-baby jeans. As tempting as it is now that your baby bump is shrinking, the last thing your healing body needs is extra friction. Trousers with thick seams, like jeans, will feel very uncomfortable. And it's not just jeans I hold a grudge against in the post-partum period, but active wear too. Hot, tight and restricting, they can create a perfect environment for irritation and infection to set in. Instead, embrace loose, natural clothing to keep you cool and comfortable.

- Take sitz baths. Bathing your perineum in a perineal sitz bath (a special shallow bowl that goes on top of the toilet to bathe your bits in) or sitting in a very shallow bath are great ways to reduce swelling, relieve itching from stitches, ease pain, prevent infection and even settle down bothersome haemorrhoids. Use warm to cool (not hot) water and add Epsom or sea salts for protection from infection and healing benefits. I also recommend adding one to two drops of essential lavender oil. This is nature's antibacterial skin-soothing elixir. If you have stitches then a maximum of 20 minutes in the bath once a day is plenty. Any more and your stitches may soften. If you have no stitches and using this for pain relief, then you can take a 'sitz bath' several times a day.

- Apply a perineal spritzer. In my opinion this is an essential for any hospital bag. Perineal spritzers are full of natural ingredients to promote healing, reduce swelling and soreness, prevent infection and nourish healing tissues. You can apply them directly or spray on to a pad for relief and nourishment where you need it most. You can make up your own by mixing 50ml of witch hazel (a natural antibacterial and astringent) with 50ml of cool boiled water and adding two drops of lavender essential oil. If this seems like too much faff, there are plenty available to buy. Three of my favourites are Bottoms Up (Natural Birthing Company), Spritz for Bits (My Expert Midwife), and Perineal Mama Mist (Fat and the Moon).

Stabilise

Pelvic floor exercises may be the last thing you feel like doing after the epic event that is childbirth! But they are honestly the best thing we can do for our healing selves. As soon as you've done your first wee after your baby is born, test those muscles out. Getting your muscles to contract and relax will act like a pump to circulate blood to your injuries and promote healing, encouraging the tissues to knit together where they're needed the most.

Early post-birth pelvic floor exercises are different to those we'll do for the rest of our life. The muscles and tissues are inflamed, stretched and sometimes cut or torn. It will not be possible to achieve our best contraction right now, but we're not aiming for this in the first few weeks. We just want to send a signal from the brain, via the nerves to the muscles, and for a message to travel back up this pathway to let us know what's going on. We are healing the muscles of our birth canal and its many nerves, the deeper pelvic floor which keeps our organs high and our pelvic ring closed, and the superficial sphincter muscles which are stretched and often sore, especially if we had a catheter or are prone to haemorrhoids. So start with remembering how to stop yourself from breaking wind or stopping your flow of urine. Perform these actions (NOT when you need to go, but when you are resting). Imagine you are mid-flow and you need to stop suddenly, or you feel the urge to break wind just as the doctors come to discuss your discharge home (this embarrassingly happened to me after my first traumatic birth, when my muscles were paralysed by pain and local anesthetic!).

In the first 2–3 weeks here's what your pelvic floor exercises should entail, after which you should feel ready to move on to task 4 (page 58) and your pelvic floor exercises for life:

- Find a comfortable position lying flat on your back with your knees bent, on your tummy with your legs straight, or on your side with a pillow between your knees.

- Take a few full breaths in for a count of six and out for a count of six, so that your diaphragm moves up and down, which will encourage the pelvic floor to follow naturally with this movement (this happens automatically). This may be the first time you've had a chance to breathe fully for months, so enjoy it!

- Find the muscles which will close or clench your poo pipe, as though you're stopping wind escaping or avoiding an anal examination! Pinch the opening shut as though you are pinching the end of a straw to not let anything out, then release, relax and let it go. Try a few more breaths before going again. Repeat x10.

- Find the muscles which close or clench your pee pipe, as though you're stopping your flow of urine mid-stream (remember not to do this when you are actually peeing as that can cause a back flow and risk infection), then release, relax and let it go. Try a few more breaths before going again. Repeat x10.

Practise this up to three times a day to restore your nerve-to-muscle connection – what we physios call motor control, but you might recognise as muscle memory. Our body responds well to feedback. If you can't sense anything happening try taking a look with a mirror or feeling (with clean hands) the outside of your passageways. You should see or feel a gathering and lift of the entrance holes to your bum, vagina and bladder.

Don't worry if you feel nothing to begin with. It is very normal for your nerves and muscles to be stunned in the first few days post-birth. Within 2–3 weeks you should get a sense of what's going on. If you don't you may need some more help to continue healing and rebuilding, so ask your midwife or doctor to check that you are doing your exercises correctly. They may not be able to do an internal examination with their finger as this could increase the infection risk, but they can observe your perineum and vaginal opening to check that it is lifting up and in when you do your 'squeezes'. They can also arrange an early referral to see a women's health physiotherapist if you need one.

Rehabilitate

As soon as the pain subsides it's easy to forget about the trauma of a perineal wound, but once the skin has healed, normally at around four to six weeks, it is time to further support the recovery of its underlying muscles. Scar massage alongside pelvic floor exercises helps the perineal and pelvic floor muscles to re-model, meaning the individual fibres are pulled to where strength is needed and the muscle starts to resemble what was there before the injury.

If you haven't got there already, progress your pelvic floor exercises to task 4 (see page 58) and from six weeks treat your scar to a tender massage and stretch. This perineal massage technique is similar to one you might have used to prepare your perineum for childbirth by stretching your perineal tissue ahead of time. This is particularly important if you have scarring from previous births that will need to give and stretch again in labour. If it's a long time since your birth injury and you have never massaged your scar, have a go! You may be surprised at not only how sensitive and tight it still is, but also how it responds and improves with massage.

TASK 6 PERINEAL MASSAGE, HOW-TO GUIDE

You can start this scar work daily from six weeks after birth, as soon as the scar has healed.

KIT YOU WILL NEED: A natural oil, such as coconut, vitamin E or even olive oil. For some self-care luxury treat yourself to Nessa Organics' Vagina Victory Oil or Natural Birthing Company's Pure Bliss.

It's best to try this in the bathroom with one foot up on the toilet seat or edge of the bath. If your scar is on one side (often episiotomy scars are on the right) ensure the same side foot is up so as to give the scar a little stretch and so that you can reach it more easily. If your partner, midwife or friend is helping you with this then lying on the bed with just one pillow is best. Try to make yourself as relaxed, comfortable and warm as possible. If you are at ease you will find it more comfortable to work on your body and go with the stretches. After a warm bath or shower is great as heat helps our tissues to stretch.

STEP 1

Gently and caringly massage the oil or balm over and around the area. Using a flat hand and gentle pressure, massage in a sweeping or circular motion. Moving and nourishing the skin on and around the scar will help to desensitise the painful bits, meaning you are more ready for the next step. Spend 1-2 minutes doing this in the early days. You'll find you can move on to step 2 more quickly as you heal.

STEP 2

Now you can get to the scar itself. Using a thumb or your first two fingers, press down into the end of your scar furthest away from your vagina with a firm pressure. There should be a strong but comfortable feeling, just on the edge of pain and soreness. Make circles with your fingers, not sliding over the scar but moving the skin and layers of tissue. Spend 30-60 seconds in this one place before moving further towards your vaginal opening and repeating. Work along your scar until you reach the vaginal opening, then work back along your scar in the opposite direction. The first few times you massage this may well be enough. Spend 2 minutes in total on this step. When you feel ready, progress to massaging at the vaginal opening itself before moving to step 3.

STEP 3

Using the pad of the thumb or first finger apply firm pressure to the entrance of your vagina, directly on to the scar. Allow the weight of your thumb or finger to weigh down on the scar, gently stretching it. Again, it should not feel painful, but just on the edge before it becomes painful. If you can tolerate it, make circles here, just as at stage 2, to mobilise the scar further. Apply pressure for around 60-90 seconds. Discomfort should settle as you massage. If it becomes painful as you work on it then it's time to stop. Give your body a few days to relax and settle before trying again.

Repeat this most days until your scar is pain free, mobile and as sensitive as the rest of the perineal tissues. Scars will change in appearance over two years, a process known as remodelling. Even if your scar is older than this and you have never worked on it, the good news is that it is still possible to change your scar tissue's elasticity and strength.

If these steps for releasing your scar still leave it feeling sore, vibrating massage tools are hugely helpful to comfortably mobilise the tissues. My regular bulk order of bullet vibrators from Love Honey always gets a raised eyebrow from whomever signs for the parcel! Sadly, the benefits are more practical than pleasurable, although I do recommend their use for both. If the scar is sore to massage or is uncomfortable in a sitting position or during sexual intercourse, I suggest you try a bullet vibrator instead of your thumb or fingers to apply pressure directly to your scar. The vibration through the scar will move the layers of tissue underneath, helping to reorganise the collagen and break down the scar tissue. It will also reduce the pain because the nerves which detect pain also detect vibration. So the brain receives messages of vibration and stretch rather than those of pain. Clever eh!

Once you have massaged and stretched your scar it's the perfect time to fire up the muscles underneath it with your pelvic floor exercises. A muscle contraction will pull along the scar and reorganise the healing muscle fibres in the direction they need to work. Just a few minutes of massage may loosen up the tissues enough for you to get your best pelvic floor contraction going. Remember you are rehabilitating your whole body – skin, muscle and joints. Birth injury healing goes deeper than we can see, into the muscle function beneath, so the combination of perineal massage and pelvic floor exercises is a winner.

Real-life story

Zoe is a mum of two, who experienced birth trauma, but fought back to full strength

We were so excited when we fell pregnant with our first child in 2015. I was lucky that my pregnancy was relatively easy with no morning sickness or nausea, no pelvic pain or any of the common pregnancy ailments. I stopped running at five months as my bump grew, but continued to swim and gained minimal weight. Overall, I wasn't too nervous about the birth. I was low risk, fit and healthy, and so planned and hoped to go as naturally as possible.

While I did have the natural birth that I had hoped for, I was pushing for over two hours and suffered a third degree tear as a result, from front to back, almost completely. We were thrilled with our gorgeous healthy boy, but I was shocked at how much pain my whole body was in. I felt like I had run a marathon and then been put into a tumble dryer on full speed for 18 hours. Every muscle ached for days and weeks.

Although it only took me a few weeks after birth to get back in my pre-pregnancy clothes and go out and about with the buggy, things didn't feel right with my body. My pelvic floor ached and I had an unusual dragging feeling. My tummy had excess loose skin and just looked totally different to before. I felt completely broken and just incredibly sad that I had taken for granted a part of me that was now so badly damaged.

Throughout the first year of my son's life I saw quite a few women's health physios. I was looking for someone who would be able to help me get back to exercise. All of them said things were 'mild' and they didn't seem to understand why I felt so symptomatic. I was prescribed Kegels and I did them religiously, but unfortunately I just didn't see the results. I wanted to get back to 'real' exercise, but lived in fear of causing myself more damage. I wanted to have more children, but was too afraid that my body wouldn't be able to cope and might tear again. I needed someone to listen to my whole story and wanted to get a true understanding of what my personal goals were.

When I saw Megan she looked at my whole body rather than just focusing 100% on the pelvic floor. She explained that although we obviously had to isolate and strengthen the pelvic floor, this was just one part of the core system and it needed to be working along with the rest of the muscles for optimum function. My perineal tear was having an effect on my posture, breathing patterns and pain throughout my body. We addressed where I was carrying muscle and released those muscles, both inside and out, and started a whole body rehab programme that targeted the weaker areas, but also incorporated the whole body's movement patterns and slowly I grew stronger.

Before long I felt confident and strong enough to try whole body weight exercises and eventually weights, all alongside my newfound pelvic floor, back and core strength. It felt *amazing* to get that muscle burn after so long without it! Nine months later I was feeling so much stronger and happier in myself, and was excited to find out I was pregnant with our second child. The knowledge and strength I had gained in my first post-natal journey put me in a totally different position for my second pregnancy. I knew so much more about my own body and how I should work with it and listen to it.

When to ask for help:

- If you feel or see your scar re-open. It is unlikely that it will be re-stitched as it's normally just the superficial skin layers and it's better to allow your body to heal naturally, but it is important to rule out an underlying infection and ensure your scar's deeper stitches remain intact.

- There is a smell, discharge or oozing from your scar that could indicate infection.

- There is a hole, gap or openness to your scar after the anticipated six-week healing time.

- Your scar is still sensitive and sore after six weeks, making sex, activity or wearing the clothes you would like to wear more difficult and uncomfortable.

- You have pain, discomfort or are struggling to open your bowels, which are all signs of constipation.

What to ask for:

- A physical examination in the first instance to ensure all is well with your body's healing.
- A swab for infection – if it's positive you will require antibiotics.
- Stool softeners or laxatives to help you poo comfortably.
- A referral to a women's health physiotherapist to support your healing and recovery.
- A referral to a perineal clinic or gynaecologist if you sustained a grade 3 or 4 tear and have not been referred already.

What's important

- Early pelvic floor exercises are not only safe, but help our healing body knit back together. Start the day you give birth, after your first wee.
- In the early days, ice packs, sitz baths and perineal spritzers will ease pain, prevent infection and promote healing. From six weeks swap these out for natural balms and oils to nourish your new tissues. Check out Naturalbirthingcompany.com, Nessaorganics.com and Myexpertmidwife.com.
- Perineal massage is not just useful prenatally, but post-natally too. Together with pelvic floor exercises you can use this to accelerate tissue repair, easing any discomfort from direct pressure and sexual intercourse.
- It is never too late to address perineal wounds and improve their flexibility, sensation and surrounding strength.

5. Abdominal birth recovery: Healing what we cannot see

Over a quarter of the babies born in the UK are delivered by Caesarean section – a cut through the lower abdominal wall. While abdominal births are common, there is still a taboo around this type of birth and many women feel ashamed or feel they need to justify how their baby was born. The method by which our babies enter the world is neither a reflection of our strength nor our capacity to deliver by other means. We all share one birth goal – that our babies arrive safely, and we are well and safe to witness it. If you do have a Caesarean I want you to know that your healing is important and your birth injuries, whether elective, emergency or somewhere in between, need just as much tender loving care as anybody else's.

The process by which our babies are born is a grey area for most mothers and no more so than an abdominal birth. As 75% of Caesarean births are unplanned, many of you reading this won't have thought much about how a Caesarean goes before you suddenly found yourself having one. Like any recovery process, the journey is much easier to follow when we understand how we got there, so here goes:

- What you can see on the outside after an abdominal birth is obviously only the skin surface. Below here are many, many layers that your doctor needs to get through before finally reaching your baby. Each of these layers will need stitches and will bear their own scar. The incision made on our skin may be curved or straight and most often lies 1-2cm above the bump of our pubic mound, often called a bikini cut. In a very few cases the surgeon may need to extend this scar to birth our baby safely and in these cases what you can see on the outside may look more like a T, J or U.

- The surgeon can then move the fascial layer, which sheathes our abdominal muscles, to one side to reach our abdominal muscles themselves. Unlike what we see on the outside, the cut made here is vertical and not horizontal, to avoid cutting across our rectus abdominis muscle. This is actually two parallel muscles and the cut goes between them, through the vertical line already formed by our linea alba (if you need a recap on anatomy see page 23), and the rectus muscle can be moved apart to reveal our uterus.

- Now the surgeon can see our uterus, but to get to our baby they need to first move our bladder and create what is affectionately called a 'bladder flap', lifting this precious organ safely away.

- The next cuts are horizontal, through the layers of our uterus to finally reach our baby.

- Amazingly, this whole process takes around five minutes from the first incision our doctor makes, but the careful repair which follows can take 45 minutes or more, as each layer is individually and meticulously stitched back together.

So what does all this mean for your recovery?

In most cases you will have been given an epidural to block your nerves from the waist down, so that you can feel no pain from the procedure. Because of this you will have had a catheter inserted into your bladder to collect urine. Both this and the manual moving of your bladder away from your womb can make peeing a little tricky after birth. It is important to check that you can pee normally before heading home. Your pain relief from surgery, immediately after birth and while still in hospital, as well as the euphoria of meeting your baby, can make you feel superhuman. Be prepared for when this wears off and don't be afraid to ask for pain relief at home if you need it.

The vertical incision at your abdominal muscle layer, while it preserves the muscles themselves, passes through the linea alba. Already thinned from pregnancy, this can struggle to heal after surgery and the two sides of the rectus abdominis muscle below the navel can remain stretched and further apart. Because of this, after the natural eight-week recovery time, a condition called diastasis rectus abdominis muscle (DRAM) is a possibility that needs to be considered. This means that the rectus abdominis muscle remains a little further apart than before your pregnancy and targeted rehabilitation is needed to strengthen and re-knit the muscles back together (more on this in chapter 8). Following a Caesarean section DRAM is most likely to be found below your tummy button, directly where your muscles were stretched, whereas following a vaginal birth DRAM is more likely to be found at and above your navel.

We cannot always predict how our births will go, but we can approach our post-natal recovery with care and attention. Our birth stories are individual to us and no two are the same. In my group of close friends nearly half of our babies (to date!) have been born abdominally. Between our small group we've seen it all; from emergency Caesareans, breach births and forceps through to pre-planned water births, surprise living room deliveries and serene elective Caesareans. While it's a unique experience, birth is birth and whole-body rehabilitation is essential for whole-body recovery both inside and out, no matter the method of delivery.

Protect

Caesarean section does not protect us from the changes our body makes through pregnancy and regardless of birth method our recovery from growing a baby needs to be considered. Our initial six to eight-week recovery is not only about our physical wounds healing, but giving our body time to heal from the stretch and strain of pregnancy. It's worth remembering, and reminding those around you and yourself, that you have undergone pregnancy, childbirth *and* major abdominal surgery. This comes with a great deal of pain, muscle and postural changes, as well as the floods of hormonal ups and downs. We need to protect our bodies and minds to encourage the healing process. The more you rest in these first few weeks the quicker your strength will return, so call on the support of those around you and share these tips with them:

- Keep using your pregnancy pillow. Not only is sleep essential for recovery, but you can use this rest time to heal in the best posture. Side-lying with a pillow between your knees to keep your pelvic bones stacked on top of one another is ideal. A pregnancy horseshoe pillow can also be wrapped around your tummy or pinch another pillow from your partner to do this job. You want to tuck this underneath your waist so that your tummy can relax fully on to it.

- Sit with support. It's tempting to hunch forward and protect a sore tummy, particularly when you have your most precious bundle curled up on your lap to coo over, but even just a few days of this will make it hard to straighten up again and your muscles will get used to this position. Try to get into a good habit straightaway or as soon as you can. Find the best chair to support your whole back while still having both feet on the floor. Use as many feeding pillows as you need underneath your little one to keep your back upright while feeding. These pillows should crucially lift your baby up to meet your breast or bottle without the need for you to slouch forwards to reach them.

- Try to minimise moving and carrying your baby. While they are still so tiny, they're already a weight that will challenge your healing body. Pain will no doubt change the way you move, lift and carry. Without even realising it your body may be subtly protecting, guarding and compensating to protect you from pain. Try not to challenge your body as it heals, which could put strain on your posture, compensatory muscles and generally make everything work much harder than it needs to at this time. Ask those around you to help out or maybe even use the pram in the house rather than carrying your baby around in the first few weeks... I know that this is easier said than done with a newborn who prefers to be with you than in their expensive buggy! It's worth a try, though, to give your body the rest it needs.

- Get prepped with older children. If this is not your first baby you may be worrying about how you will take care of older siblings. Embrace their help and set your home up so that the changes are fun for them. New steps and stools which are just for them worked great for my children after I had tummy surgery to repair a hernia. They were fighting over these to stand at the sink, get in the car or up and down from the table instead of asking me to pick them up. You can start this before your new baby arrives if you are preparing for an abdominal birth, so that they already know the drill!

- Eat and drink well to minimise inflammation and constipation. You want to support your healing with warm nutritious food and plenty of water. High-sugar, fizzy drinks and sweet snacks can lead to bloating and constipation while providing little of what you need. Of course, this can be a challenge when another life is your first priority, but your healing and wellbeing will help them to thrive. Take time to consider how to get a healthy warming meal every day, be this from calling on family, friends and neighbours or ordering in ready-made nutritious dinners.

- Start pelvic floor exercises straightaway. Yes, this is an essential first step whether your birth is vaginal or abdominal. You are helping your body recover from pregnancy, not just birth. Task 4 on page 58 is a great place to start.

Stabilise

Pain and inflammation as well as changes from pregnancy and new motherhood can take their toll on our posture. We need to activate and exercise our postural muscles early on to prevent other bigger muscles from taking over, especially following abdominal birth. Both the stretch of pregnancy and the surgical Caesarean incision can reduce not only the strength in the muscles of our abdominal cylinder, but also our ability to find it and work it. Restoring your flexibility and doing muscle activation exercises will benefit not only your posture but your everyday movement as well. While you need to rest from structured exercise until six to eight weeks after abdominal birth, task 7 provides the strength and stretch training you need to stabilise while protecting your healing. Stick with this and pelvic floor tasks 3 (see page 55) and 4 (see page 58) until that six to eight-week mark when your scar has healed.

TASK 7 STRETCH AND STRENGTH AFTER SURGERY

Following any abdominal surgery it is totally normal to feel a little tug when you start to move, but this should not be painful. You need to encourage your body to stretch and tug a little to desensitise the scar tissue and that way, bit by bit, you will be able to stretch further, and do more and more without any pain at all.

It is safe to start these exercises as soon as you feel ready. They are no more challenging than lifting and carrying your new baby. You must wait six to eight weeks before returning to a full exercise program, but you can work on these most days until then.

KIT YOU WILL NEED: A soft Pilates ball to squeeze between your knees (you can use a cushion if you don't have one).

Cat circles:

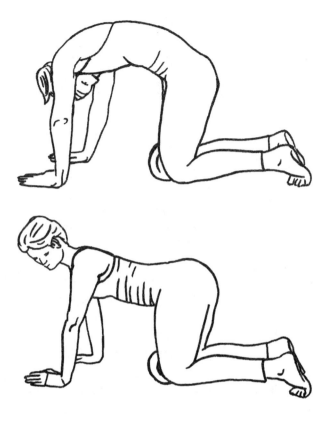

This is a great way to gently move and stretch your tummy and your new scar. On your hands and knees hold a ball between your thighs to activate your inner thigh and other pelvic muscles. Make exaggerated circular movements with your pelvis. Start with your whole body rounded, chin on your chest, your tail tucked under as though you are trying to look inside your belly button. Now keep everything else the same and push your bottom back to the right. Release your tail and arch your back, lifting your head up and out as you move your hips through the middle to the left. Let your tummy fall away to the floor to a comfortable stretch. As you circle back and around to the right pick up your tummy, round your back once more and return your chin to your chest to completely round the body and come back to your start position. Move as though you are using your tail to draw a big circle on the wall behind you. Complete a few circles in this direction before changing. Do this for 2-4 minutes.

High keeling heel press:

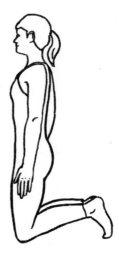

Kneeling is a great position to reset your posture, straighten up your spine, and activate your tummy and your pelvic floor. Grow as tall as you can in this position, lifting the crown of your head and your breastbone towards the ceiling, imagine you have on your favourite necklace and you are showing it off to the room. Press your heels firmly together and notice your bottom tighten and push your hips forwards, giving your tummy a little stretch. Hold this position and heel squeeze for 10 seconds. Relax. Repeat x6. Next add an overhead arm movement to further work your tummy, and open up your chest and back. Breathe out as you raise your arms overhead and inhale as you lower them. Throughout the movement maintain your heel squeeze and keep your best posture. You should feel your tummy tighten as your arms go up and loosen as your arms come down. Repeat for 2 minutes.

Overhead arms at wall:

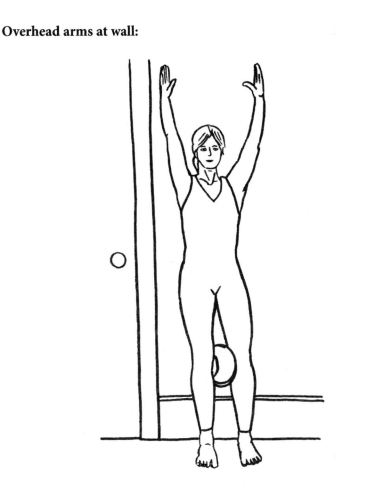

Stand with your feet a little away from a wall, hold the ball between your knees and lean your back into the wall. Take your time here to straighten up and lengthen your spine. When you're ready, press your back into the wall to create a flat spine. On your exhale hold it here as you take your arms up and over your head. Inhale and lower your arms. Feel your tummy draw in and up gently as you work to hold your back against the wall. Repeat for 2–4 minutes.

In the first few weeks post-birth to stabilise your healing tummy and support your posture it can also be helpful to add in belly taping or a splint. Much like casting a broken bone, we can stabilise our tummy to encourage healing of the skin and knitting back together of the muscles underneath with external strapping. But remember, just like the cast, it is not this tool which does the healing, it just creates a more stable environment for that to happen. Your rehabilitation exercises are what restores your abdominal cylinder muscle strength; a tummy splint just supports its action. There are many 'post-baby belts' on the market, but the simplest are the best. In the absence of separation of your tummy muscles (DRAM or diastasis recti abdominis muscle) you're just looking to encourage the up and inwards support that your deep muscle corset normally provides. Cross over straps are therefore the best as they mimic the muscle pull across your midline. You don't need it too tight, just enough to give your muscles the support to work when they're needed. It's best to avoid true 'binders' that promise to cinch or 'enhance' your waist. It might sound good, but these circular bandages can create too much pressure, which has to go somewhere, and more often than not this is down on the pelvic floor. Already weakened by pregnancy, any added pressure from above is not welcome on a post-partum bladder, bowel and pelvic floor muscles. Likewise, clothing that pulls in too tight around your middle should be avoided for several weeks to prevent tightening your tummy beyond what it can tolerate and shifting the pressure 'down below'.

If you'd like to try an effective strap see task 14 on page 170 . This is a taping strategy I use often to provide stability and support after abdominal birth.

Rehabilitate

Beyond the six to eight-week healing period immediately after a Caesarean section, an abdominal birth recovery is similar to that of a vaginal birth in all aspects, apart from that scar below your knicker line. You need to approach your pelvic floor, abdominal and pelvic ring rehabilitation pragmatically. While it is tempting to skip past these other sections, hopeful that your pelvic floor was preserved by not giving birth vaginally, it is often pregnancy and not the manner in which you give birth that challenges your body and its strength the most. Review task 4 on page 58 to check your pelvic floor strength. If this is a challenge then this is the best task for you to start your rehabilitation with.

Abdominal activation like that in task 12 (see page 157) is great for not only healing DRAM, but also recovery following pregnancy and particularly an abdominal birth. By finding, feeling and exercising each layer of tummy muscle we can not only rebuild strength but also enhance our recovery and aid the scar formation. When we move our tissues the way they were intended scars pull flatter and become less visible. Make task 12 your next step in rehabilitation from six to eight weeks and once your scar has healed, in order to reset your abdominal muscles sequencing.

Something that is unique to your recovery after a Caesarean compared to a vaginal birth is your abdominal scar. While it is hidden most of the time, you can't ignore it. You need that scar to heal well to restore your low abdominal muscle tone and strength, prevent scar thickening and return normal sensations – the aim is not only to be pain free, but to replace numbness with full sensitivity and prevent the dreaded 'apron' pouching. Women often complain of this 'bulging' over their scar and altered sensitivity for months if not years following abdominal birth. Scar massage is the first step to improving both these complaints. As Caesarean recovery is not given the voice that it should have and scars are often hidden through fear of shaming, it can be hard to access the advice, technique and strategy to do this well. So here it is, step by step, so you can heal and nurture your new *birthmark*, feel connected to it and acknowledge it with pride.

TASK 8 ABDOMINAL SCAR MASSAGE

From six to eight weeks, providing there has been no set back in scar healing, you can begin scar massage. A friend, partner or massage therapist can help you with this if you need support, but you'll soon be ready to try for yourself.

KIT YOU WILL NEED: A natural oil, such as coconut, vitamin E, almond or jojoba oil. You could also treat yourself to Pure Bliss (Natural Birthing Company) or a nourishing balm such as Nessa's Scar Saviour (Nessa Organics).

This whole routine should take no more than 3–5 minutes.

STEP 1

Sweep around your tummy with the flat of your hand, avoid your scar itself and just massage over your tummy. The scar will stretch gently as you move all of the connective tissues around it. The only rule is to go in a clockwise direction to follow the movement of your bowel. Using your oil or balm as you do this makes it feel more comfortable, as well as nourishing your post-pregnancy tummy.

STEP 2

Using the pad of one or two fingers, trace along the scar, just above it. Press down firmly enough to move the skin and scar in small circles. You're looking for a strong stretchy sensation, but not pain. Work along the scar like this, moving it in a circular motion. As you come back the other way massage again in circles, but now just below your scar. It may surprise you to feel tension either side of your scar itself, but remember the multiple layers beneath your fingers that have been involved in birthing your baby.

STEP 3

Now try the same thing on the scar itself, moving the scar in a circular direction one way, then in the opposite direction as you come back along the scar. With firm pressure, spend extra time on bumpy, tighter spots. It's completely normal for the scar and skin around it to become red. This is a sign that fresh blood has been drawn to the area, which is essential for remodelling the tissues, but the scar should not weep, stay red or be more painful afterwards. After six to eight weeks, and providing there has been no infection or re-opening of your scar over this time, then your tissues will already be healed and knitted back together, so there is very little risk of your scar re-opening and this gentle massage will help remodel the underlying tissues, so that your scar is softer and less visible.

STEP 4

Finish by stretching and moving the new tissue along the lines of stress. For the tummy this means up and down. We want the new tissue fibres to organise themselves straight up and down, so pull on the skin around the scar up and down. Feel a strong, comfortable stretch, and work along the scar area in both directions. Give your tummy a few gentle loving sweeps of oil or balm to finish. Make this part of your self-care routine to reconnect and heal.

If it is too sore, too sensitive, or indeed too numb then try this with a little vibration tool. Again our trusty bullet vibrator works wonders to mobilise scar tissue, relieve pain and improve sensation. Use the tool instead of your fingers to comfortably get deeper into your scar tissue.

Real-life story

Fran is the mother of two boys and a strong, cold-water swimmer

My first baby was in an undiagnosed stargazing position, meaning his back was against my back and he was looking out at the world. I was more than two weeks overdue, and was dragged kicking and screaming into an induction. After more than 12 hours on the induction drip (and no pain relief... what was I thinking?) I was only at 9cm and my son's heart rate became erratic, so I had an emergency C-section. My pelvic floor had taken a bashing and I had both the challenges of an almost vaginal birth and an abdominal birth to consider.

Two and a half years later I had the opposite trauma of a birth that lasted 54 minutes from first contraction to my son flying out like a Tic Tac... My pelvic floor was desperately in need of some TLC.

Fifteen months on I began to experience symptoms of pelvic floor prolapse. I had been confident I was OK, but I soon realised I was wrong when after long periods standing up I'd feel as though I had a full tampon working its way out of me, even though I wasn't using one! I'd experienced urine leaks after emptying my bladder and forget running after my small children – my pelvic floor couldn't handle it at all.

I took myself off to a physiotherapist – Megan! – and found out that it wasn't just my pelvic floor that was struggling, but my first birth had left my core weak. After learning what was wrong I felt confident that I could lessen my symptoms and reverse some of them, but I had a lot of work to do. After a few one-on-one sessions I found and could use my tummy muscles, and then graduated to classes in addition to my homework rehab. The plan was simple: by building up all the muscles that work with my pelvic floor I would put less pressure on the floor itself, especially when working my front abdominals – which was handy, because when I started, thanks to my C-section, mine couldn't even perform a crunch without spitting my vagina out! I had already used a couple of gadgets to help work my pelvic floor, but Megan added a pelvic floor toner to the routine, which worked all of my muscles together and she told me to use it at least three times a week – long enough to experience muscle fatigue or it wouldn't be effective. I learnt how to mentally cue my pelvic floor to give it a head start before movements that would put it under stress and, while I still sometimes have to mentally cue the darn thing, some of the time it's now automatic. I can happily plank, crunch, curl and generally feel stronger than I ever have in my life. We can't stop traumatic births if they happen, but we don't have to live with the symptoms of damage afterwards.

When to ask for help:

- Your scar becomes increasingly painful, thickened, numb or overly sensitive. While this is expected in the first eight weeks, it should settle and become easier with time. If it's not changing or your levels of discomfort are increasing then do ask for help.

- You can see bulging below your navel, popping out of your midline or indentations that could indicate DRAM (abdominal muscle separation).

What to ask for:

- Some massage therapists, as well as some women's health physiotherapists, are specialists in scar massage if you need some help with this. You may have to self-fund your treatment, but your doctor should be able to suggest where to go.

- Silicone strips are recommended to reduce excessive scarring and minimise scar appearance once the healing has occurred. These are applied directly to a scar after the normal six to eight-week recovery time, for a minimum of 12 hours a day over three months. Internationally, this is considered the first-line management for raised, sore or thickened scars… Yes, I agree, every mother with a Caesarean scar should be given these at their six-week check-up. Why aren't we? Your guess is as good as mine. But at least we now know to ask for them! And if you have to self-fund them yourself you can expect to pay around £30 for strips that can be washed and reused, and will last the three months if you look after them well. If you can afford to, these are 100% worth the investment in my opinion.

What's important

- Your body needs to recover and restore itself following pregnancy, regardless of the type of birth you experienced. Beyond your initial six to eight-week recovery from abdominal surgery your post-natal rehabilitation should include the rehabilitation of your tummy, pelvis and pelvic floor, just like a vaginal birth.
- Abdominal births are much more common than you might think. Don't be afraid to talk about your story and needs.
- Protect your healing body by adopting your best posture straightaway.
- Stabilise with early pelvic floor exercises. Yes, really. Pregnancy is as much a stress on the pelvic floor as delivery.
- Begin scar massage as soon as healing has taken place, usually six to eight weeks after you gave birth.

6. Prolapse: The silent epidemic

If you've never heard of pelvic organ prolapse, you'll probably skim-read this section thinking 'Crikey! That sounds awful. I hope that never happens to me.' This is what I thought. In fact, more accurately and rather smugly, I thought, 'That's never going to happen to me. I'm a physiotherapist' – until three weeks after my first baby was born...

My story

Two days after my waters slowly broke at home (less of a tide, more of a trickle), and after having no contractions, I underwent an induction. I had already decided that I didn't want an epidural and I stuck to this even as the induction drugs kicked in and my labour pains sent me into a hypnotic, spaced out state. In hindsight I can see that, given the circumstances, things may have been easier if I had been more open to change. I had a wonderful midwife and I remember her saying to me, 'You can have an epidural anytime you want. Just say the word. I'll make it happen.' I trusted her completely and knew that she would, but I wanted to do this hard thing on my own, although I hadn't considered that with syntocinon pumping through my body via a drip I was already under medical management and far from 'on my own' in this battle. So, 12 hours later, epidural-less but now high on pethidine, the hard miles were still ahead. After two hours of pushing I knew things weren't going well. From being insistent that I give birth on all fours to protect my perineum and catch my baby myself I now found myself on my back, legs in stirrups, with a doctor between my legs who muttered to my midwife, 'If I don't cut her she's going to tear.'

Up until this point the worst thing that I thought could happen to me was a perineal tear. Prolapse was still not even factored into my vision of my post-natal recovery. I was feeling strong through my pregnancy, lifting weights right up until week 40, but what I hadn't thought about was that I had also built a strong and consequently stiff pelvic floor and perineum, that struggled to 'give' when my baby appeared. The hours I had spent stretching and in ante-natal yoga were perhaps not enough. I had found my own self-care far more difficult to prioritise than caring for others. When I see women in my clinic in the run-up to their labour to teach them perineal massage, I am still a little embarrassed that I struggled to do this on myself, clouded by my misbelief that pelvic floor trauma does not happen to a pelvic floor physiotherapist.

In the delivery room, through a haze, I instructed the doctor where I wanted my episiotomy to protect my nether regions and demanded I was told when to pant my baby out. The medical staff nodded politely, but had the ventouse cup – a plunger-like instrument that goes inside your vagina to clasp the baby's head and pull him or her down the birth canal – ready. Mothers who are induced are more likely to need some help, such as ventouse or even forceps, delivering the baby's head, as we are confined to a bed and unable to use 'active birth' positions and gravity to help our baby drop down. With the induction drip in situ and often an epidural too it can feel harder, if not impossible, to push at the last hurdle.

I may have delivered Robyn vaginally, but I don't refer to her birth as a natural delivery, because it was a medical one, with doctors performing a 'slash and grab' to help her out. After the birth, I found myself watching my husband cooing over our baby, pretending to ignore the drama happening between my legs as the medical team struggled to repair the damage of a tear, episiotomy and ventouse delivery.

Like most new mothers I was excited to take my baby home and prioritised her needs over my own. I was determined to continue to demonstrate what I thought was 'strength'. At the time I thought being strong meant doing it all on my own. My husband was back at work within a couple of days and our parents headed home after cuddles, so doing it on my own was a badge of honour. I now feel I was misguided. I needed to heal and I needed help. I can see that I should have found the strength to follow all my own advice, insisted friends and family came to support me, and invested more time in my own healing. I needed to take the load off my nether regions, take sitz baths and receive healing massage to ease my body – which felt like it had been hit by a bus. I needed to eat nourishing meals that had been lovingly prepared for me and to nap when I could.

But this is really about what came next. After four weeks I had healed enough to brave a longer walk than our new daily routine of a lap of the block. I set out to visit my old work colleagues and show off my baby girl in her buggy, but half-way there I noticed things were not feeling right between my legs and I couldn't wait to get home to examine myself. Hands shaking, I found a mirror, lay back on my bed and ventured down there. Nothing. I could see nothing, yet when I stood up I could feel the pressure of my vaginal walls caving in on one another. I was constantly aware of my vagina, which was very hard to explain. It wasn't pain as such, but a constant discomfort, like a tampon had moved out of place or I was wearing knickers that were a little too tight. I now realise my pelvic organs weren't supported. There was too much movement and the walls were effectively rubbing against one another, but still on examination things felt relatively 'normal'. Confused and desperate to understand what had happened to my body I booked myself in with a treasured colleague from the London Women's Centre, Demetri Panayi. My physio friends have since asked if I was embarrassed being examined by a surgeon I work with professionally. I felt anything but – Demetri was the only person I would have felt comfortable with as I trust his judgement completely and I was ready to learn how to fix this. He examined me in a standing position, something I couldn't do myself, which confirmed my worst fears: both an anterior and posterior vaginal wall prolapse. It was mild and only present in standing, but it was there. And I spent the next two years distracted by it, being my own professional case study and rehabilitating, literally from the ground up.

So if you too think this couldn't happen, or if this is you and you're screaming, 'Yes! Yes, that's it! That's how I feel!' please read on, because the most important thing you need to know is you can fix this.

Pelvic organ prolapse is the downward movement of the bladder, womb or bowel into our vaginal space. It feels like something taking up the space inside your vagina; a sensation of rubbing or pressure between your vaginal walls; a tampon falling out of place; a dragging, heavy or bulging sensation down there. This happens when the muscle of the vaginal wall and the ligaments supporting it have been overstretched and slackened, creating space for the pelvic organs above to move into. In the absence of prolapse the pelvic organs sit above the hammock of the pelvic floor and are supported by its many muscles. The passages from the bladder, womb and bowel leading to these organs are relatively vertical and dependent on the muscular walls of the vagina and pelvic floor to hold their shape and position. This is perhaps an evolutionary error – if these passageways were horizontal (like most other mammals) our pelvic floors would not be susceptible to the effects of gravity and this chapter would be irrelevant!

The symptoms of a pelvic organ prolapse vary depending on the type and severity of the injury. There are several degrees of pelvic organ prolapse,

Different Types of Prolapse

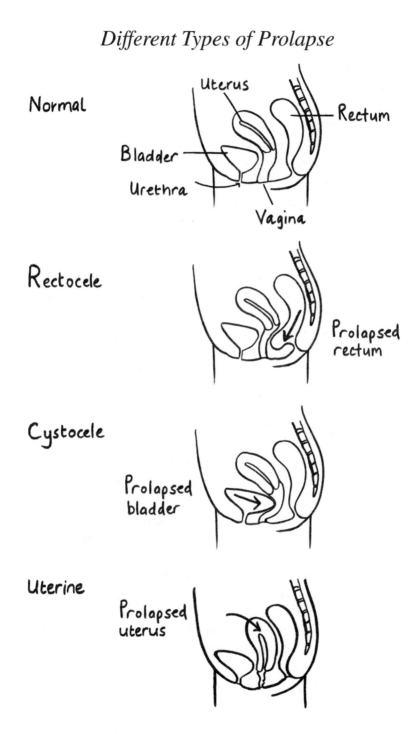

Normal

Uterus

Rectum

Bladder

Urethra

Vagina

Rectocele

Prolapsed rectum

Cystocele

Prolapsed bladder

Uterine

Prolapsed uterus

ranging from 1-2, which is mild to moderate, through to 3-4, which is severe. But please don't let this worry you. In women of child-bearing age it's very rare to suddenly find yourself at 4. Most women I see are grade 1 or 2. Many are unaware that they even have pelvic organ prolapse and the majority can be completely rehabilitated. In some there may be a prolapse of just one organ, such as the bladder and this is called a cystocele. Or there can be movement, displacement and prolapse of more than one organ at a time. A cystocele can occur with or without a rectocele (back wall prolapse) or uterine prolapse. Each can be independent of the other and comes with their own symptoms, worries and fears. Similarly, their rehabilitation is unique too.

Cystocele

When the front wall of the vagina and pelvic floor are weakened, the bladder and/or urethra push into the vaginal space. This sort of prolapse is most likely to occur after childbirth and up to a third of women who experience traumatic births, such as my first experience, will sustain an injury to their anterior vaginal wall, which may result in either a urethrocele or cystocele or both.

You may notice a pink balloon shape at your vaginal opening. This is likely be your bladder and this is called a cystocele. With a bladder prolapse symptoms of leaking urine for seemingly no reason or when you exert yourself, such as coughing or sneezing, are likely. But you may also notice urgency about going for a wee as the bladder has less space to fill, or that you are unable to fully empty your bladder as the bladder neck or its urethra is kinked like a hosepipe. In some cases it's this tube which carries urine from the bladder that is sitting too low and not the bladder itself. This is called a urethrocele and in my experience can cause women the most discomfort down there. This is because the urethra sits right inside the vaginal opening, where all the sensory nerves lie. You're very likely to be aware of this prominent organ when you move, cough or sneeze as it's sitting lower than its original position. You may even be able to see the round opening of your 'pee pipe', especially if you've had a catheter or any injury to the urethral sphincter muscles, the ones which keep it closed tight. When the urethra sits lower than the pelvic hammock it can be irritated by your underwear and/or movement. Exertion can also cause urine to pass down and out. This means you're likely to be constantly aware of this mild prolapse, and have increased risk of urinary infections and wet knickers, all of which makes it very uncomfortable down there.

Rectocele

When the back wall of the vagina is thinned, overstretched or weak the rectum can push forwards into the vaginal passage. This is called a rectocele. The back muscle is often injured when there is a perineal tear in childbirth or when an episiotomy – a cut through the back pelvic floor muscle on one side to create space for the baby or babies –is performed. Chronic constipation can also lead to posterior wall prolapse as the wall is repeatedly strained by heavy stools and forceful expulsion. You may be able to see or feel the ridged soft posterior wall ballooning into your vaginal space. This new space is convenient for poo to sit in and become hard, giving you the frustrating feeling of needing to open your bowels, but being unable to go. Or you may experience the opposite: a sudden need to go to the loo, because the muscles at your rectum and anus are stretched and weakened, and unable to hold as much or for as long as they once could. This can also result in leaking urine as the rectocele pushes up against the urethra and bladder, especially when the rectum is full of poo. Some women have to push the rectocele up with their hands to poo or support their perineum holding tissue up against themselves to stop it giving too much when they open their bowels. You may recognise and relate to this – it's one of the reasons us physios talk about poo a lot, and making the stools softer and easier to pass is step one in protecting this injury from any further overstretch and strain (see pages 200–202 on making pooing easier).

Uterine prolapse

When any part of the pelvic floor structure is weakened or injured, there is a risk of a uterine prolapse. The uterus (womb) and cervix sit bang in the middle of the pelvic floor hammock and an injury anywhere in the hammock can mean that the uterus sits lower to the ground. This feels like the typical dragging or heaviness associated with pelvic organ prolapse. Women often tell me, 'I feel like I'm being turned inside out' or 'Everything is falling out.' You may be able to see or feel your cervix within your vaginal space, which means it will be uncomfortable when you're standing or carrying any extra load, such as your baby. It may be difficult to use tampons as your vaginal space is taken up, which can also make sexual intercourse uncomfortable and sometimes painful.

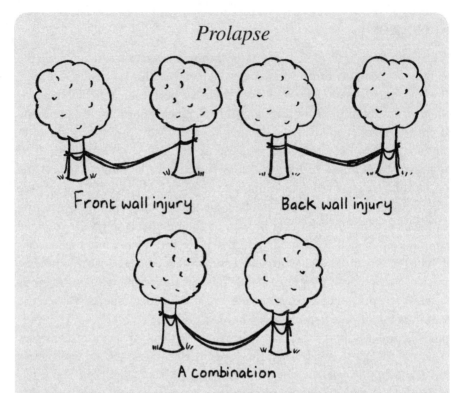

Prolapse

Front wall injury

Back wall injury

A combination

Normal: I often use a hammock analogy to best explain what's happening: strong and stable trees (our pelvic joints), stiff ropes (ligaments and tendons between the bones and connecting our muscles to our bones) and taut fabric (our pelvic floor muscle) make the pelvic organs well supported and comfortable in their hammock.

Anterior wall injury: An overstretch or injury to the front of the pelvic floor and its ropes means everything sits a bit lower and falls to the front. Our bladder and/or it's urethral tube can fall down, sit lower or just feel very uncomfortable. If the pelvic joint trees become wobbly then this will result in similar symptoms, much like in the presence of symphysis pubis dysfunction (SPD).

Posterior wall injury: The back rope becomes stretched, frayed, thin and less supportive, dragging the pelvic floor and consequently the pelvic organs lower at the back. If the pelvic joints are open or moving too much, then it's the equivalent of the back tree constantly swaying, giving little stability and stillness to the pelvic floor hammock.

Perineal body injury: This can occur slowly over time with repetitive overstrain from strenuous sports or tasks, constipation, coughing and pregnancy. These are all load-bearing challenges, which create stress and which our pelvic floor muscles, and its tendons, may not yet be strong enough to support and withstand. As a result, the fabric of the hammock becomes stretched and thinned. This can also happen with trauma, including forceps delivery, tears or an episiotomy during birth. The pelvic floor organs are no longer supported high above the ground, and the hammock, it's ropes and trees need more support or, better still, more strength.

So much pelvic floor rehabilitation focus is given to the muscular hammock, with little consideration to the trees, without which there is no hammock. Most of us take the sturdy supportive nature of our pelvis for granted. If the pelvis is unstable, moving too much, painful or compromised, then the actions and supportive nature of the pelvic floor hammock will be compromised too. A hammock cannot carry any load without first having a stable base. Sometimes the hammock is totally fine, with good muscle bulk and tension, but it is the trees, the pelvic ring joints, which are moving too much, stretched and unsupportive.

Any form of prolapse is a demonstration of injury, overstretch and laxity, and so a combination of types may be present.

Hypermobility

Pelvic organ prolapse is a hyper-mobile injury, which means things are moving too much. Something similar happens in pregnancy and birth, because all our body's structures are moved and stretched to their limit, so healing and rebuilding after pregnancy and birth is all about correcting this. To reduce the amount of movement taking place, we need to stabilise the trees, re-tie that hammock and repair the fabric, and then we can carry any load we need.

Approximately 5% of us have one or more hypermobile joints. Hypermobility syndrome is a diagnosis given to those of us who are super-bendy or double-jointed. Hyper means more and mobility means movement. Those of us with hypermobility are likely to have a stretchier type of collagen or connective tissue that is more lax than others. It's just part of our genetic makeup and often hereditary. While *more movement* sounds good and something most of us feel we need, especially when attempting to keep up in yoga class, it turns out being really bendy isn't so great after having children, and it can become a concern and even a problem. The mechanical and hormonal changes of our childbearing years stretch our bodies unrecognisably, putting extra strain on the ligaments and muscles which hold our bony skeleton together, and if coupled with hypermobility this can result in overstretch, joint injury and even pelvic organ prolapse. With a pelvis that moves more it is understandable that our pelvic floor and the organs it supports move more too. Hypermobility syndrome is considered a significant risk factor for pelvic organ prolapse, pelvic floor dysfunction and pelvic pain. While we cannot change our genetic makeup, we can recognise the increased risk and protect our bodies from extra stretch and strain. If you have been diagnosed with or suspect that you are hypermobile, pay particular attention to the Protect and Stabilise sections in this and all chapters as your body needs a little bit more cradling, support and defence.

Protect

Knowledge is the first step in protecting the pelvic floor from what it's not yet ready to cope with. Hopefully you now know that those minor leaking incidents are not 'normal mishaps', but could be clues to a greater injury that you shouldn't ignore. Unlike what you see on those cringy bladder weakness adverts, incontinence is not normal. It can be a sign of a much more substantial injury and the earlier you act the better. If you have any of the signs of pelvic organ prolapse (weakness, urgency, bulging, discomfort, pain, heaviness...) then your first job is to visit your GP and ask for an examination. Clearly, confirmation (or not) of what you're dealing with is essential for starting the process of healing and rebuilding.

Your second job is to take a step back so that you can take a good long look at what is happening. Caught in the middle of life you may have taught yourself not to listen to your body or take note when it shouts out, instead opting for a pad to dull the noise, soak up the leaks or ignore the pain. It's a good idea to take stock of when you feel your symptoms and notice what's occurring in your body, to your body or within your life at that moment. Is it always a certain time of day or only with particular activities? Is it when you go to the toilet, are feeling tired or stressed or after sex?

Here are my tips on listening to your body and responding appropriately in order to protect and heal:

- Reduce the amount of time you spend in activities which bring on your symptoms and modify these to lessen the strain. If they're big tasks then break them up throughout the day, so that your body has time to rest between challenges. Stick to when you feel your prolapse the least, so that it can heal. Protect and limit problematic activities now and you will heal and build the strength to cope with more. Keep pushing on despite a prolapse and you may find that things start to feel a little worse. Always increase your activity slowly after pregnancy and childbirth, just as you would after any injury.

- Modify physical exercise. It might be a good idea to opt out of exercise that leaves you more uncomfortable while you heal and strengthen, and allow yourself to get comfortable with working at a lower intensity. If you leak when you run, have to frequently dash off to the bathroom at dance class or feel heavy after gym then these activities are probably not doing your pelvic floor much good. You can re-introduce these activities slowly when you feel stronger and, in the meantime, find activities that are not symptomatic (bring on your symptoms).

- Avoid straining and constipation. You want a stool to enter the vicinity of your pelvic floor when it is ready to be expelled, not sit there heavy, stretching and straining the muscles of your back wall.

- Try and get into a healthy bladder habit where you go every three to four hours. Relax on the toilet and fully empty so that you can fully refill. Going 'just in case' or little and often might be tempting, but the last thing you need in addition to pelvic organ prolapse is a sensitive bladder that needs to empty hourly!

- Set a goal to be within 5kg of your pre-baby weight and make a plan to get there (if you're not there already), but be careful to follow the advice in this book about returning to exercise. Weight gain is one of the main risk factors for pelvic organ prolapse and while this is unavoidable in pregnancy (10-15kg is expected and very normal), returning to a healthy weight is beneficial not just for your vagina, but for your cardiovascular health too.

- Address any low back or pelvic pain with treatment, manual therapy or rehabilitation. Remember the 'trees' are as important as the 'hammock'. Tasks 2 (see page 39), 10 (see page 140) and 11 (see page 143) should all be ticked off as part of your prolapse rehabilitation.

For me, after my first baby the activity which left me most uncomfortable was wearing her in a sling. This was something I imagined I would do endlessly, yet I found myself struggling with pain and heaviness in my vagina if I allowed myself more than 30 minutes of 'baby-wearing' at a time. So I only did it for 30 minutes and as the months went on, even when I was tempted to do more, I stuck to it. Although my strength was building, so was my baby's weight. She was no longer the size of a newborn or sitting peacefully in a sling, so while it was tempting to feel that I should be going for longer in order to progress, I was progressing by increasing the weight I was carrying instead – my daughter was helping me grow stronger just through her own beautiful development!

After I had my second baby I stuck a spreadsheet to the fridge door to keep check of the amount of time I spent on my feet. This helped me to plan my day and gradually increase the load or pressure on my pelvic floor. I knew that two 40-minute round trips to and from my older daughter's nursery in one day would be too much for my post-natal body, so I walked to drop off and drove to pick up. Gradually I introduced walking both ways and soon I could also add a walk, shop or other activity into my day too. While these activities might seem anything but strenuous before having a baby, don't underestimate the challenge they may present afterwards and build them up slowly. Rest and activity modification won't do the healing on their own, but they will protect you from continuous movement so that the muscles have a stable base from which to work from and heal.

Asking for help, taking time out to heal and putting ourselves first are not signs of weakness, and there are no medals handed out for taking on too much too soon. If it helps, think of your body not as your own but as your best friend's. She's shared a secret with you that she's afraid she has a prolapse. She feels too embarrassed, too tired and too overwhelmed to take it all in and get to grips with the rehabilitation. Wouldn't you cradle her baby for a while? Take her by the hand to her GP to seek all of the help and support she deserves? Provide encouragement with her rehabilitation and meal planning, so that she heals and nourishes her body? Now take that advice for your own body.

Stabilise

If we think of pelvic organ prolapse like a broken arm, then this stabilise phase is like wearing a cast on the healing bones. The cast keeps everything in place so that the bones can mend and knit back together. If we were to remove the cast and shake our arm around, then this will once more move the bony ends apart and all that knitting and mending goes back to square one. While the cast doesn't do the healing, it creates the best environment for our body to do the work. It's the same for the pelvic floor. We must provide the most ideal environment for healing with our best posture, exercise that promotes stability and 'casts' in the form of pessaries if we need them.

Our posture is key to how our pelvic floor feels. Remember how the pelvic floor buckles and slackens if you tuck your bottom underneath you? Maybe you only feel your prolapse after lounging in your favorite soft chair or reclining on a sun lounger – activities that feel 'restful' – but what happens to your pelvis in these positions is that when your tail is tucked under, all your weight is on your sacrum and your pelvic floor becomes lax. Coming out of these positions you can feel uncomfortable and heavy down there, despite feeling as though you've been taking the load off. Instead, try and get into a habit of carrying 'good' posture in sitting, standing and even when relaxed. Use the cue 'stand (or sit) tall'. Imagine lengthening from the top of your head, as though there's a thread coming out from your centre parting and that thread is being pulled up towards the ceiling. When you're sitting or lying, try holding a Pilates ball between your knees to keep your tummy muscles occupied, and stop you rolling back or crossing your legs (something I'm often guilty of).

When you're standing, try taking one step forward to share your weight between your front and back leg. It's much harder to slouch or drop a hip in this position than when your feet are in parallel. Perfecting your posture is never more important than when you do your pelvic floor exercises. These are essential for creating stability and are the first line of treatment for pelvic organ prolapse (if you skipped tasks 1 and 2 flick back to the first steps for prolapse recovery on pages 30–39). They can feel tough to do when the pelvic floor is moving too much and feeling out of place, so we need to take things slowly, without the challenges of gravity or even having to hold our posture unsupported. Lying on our tummy is great as this not only takes the load off, but lifts our tailbone, setting our pelvic floor in its best position for the task. If this isn't comfortable for you, lying on your back is fine, just make sure your back isn't squashed into the bed. Only once you feel ready and are growing stronger can you start to add your first load – gravity – but this is still just the foundations of the strength you will need to heal a pelvic organ prolapse. Once you can do tasks 4 and 5 on pages 58–67, you are then ready for task 9 on page 118: raising the floor.

Pessaries are great

Alongside pelvic floor exercises, let's talk about pessaries. These are medical devices inserted into the vagina to support our pelvic organs where the muscles are struggling to. Pessaries act like shelves for the pelvic organs; they give the fabric of the hammock a second layer. Imagine putting a second hammock on top of the one that you have, so that the load of gravity and everything above it is shared between the pelvic floor muscles and the pessary.

Pessaries work in two ways:

- A pessary stabilises the pelvic floor muscles so that it can repair and protect us from any further injury. Many are worn only when we are loading or putting pressure on our pelvic floor, such as during a run or exercise class, subsequent pregnancies or to enable us to manage everyday tasks. They brace the muscles like scaffolding, so that we can continue to engage in what we enjoy without fear of damage or impeding our recovery. If by the end of the day you are more aware of your prolapse symptoms or 'you're fine unless…' then you may benefit from a pessary alongside rehabilitation to restore your strength. The goal would be to wear a pessary for as long as you need it. This may be until you have had sufficient time to rehabilitate or when the pressures on your pelvic floor return to 'normal' – in other words you have given birth.

- A pessary also puts everything where it needs to be to function. The pelvic floor has to work really hard to return prolapse back to its normal position. We are asking an already challenged muscle to perform an incredible task – to lift everything back up and in. But if we use a pessary to lift our prolapse up and in, then our muscles only have to work on holding it there. The pessary does the lifting into the correct position and you can start your strengthening there, making a seemingly impossible task more achievable. Once you have built strength enough for the pelvic floor to hold this position on its own, the pessary can be removed.

Pessaries come in all sorts of wonderful shapes and sizes, because so do we. There is an array of rings, cubes, sponges and discs that either fill up your vaginal space or sit snugly deep inside your body at the neck of your womb. There are big ones, small ones and every size in between, and the size of the device is not a measure of the size of your vagina, but the inside of your bony pelvis, which is almost impossible to measure. It may take several goes to find the right size and shape to suit your body. This does not mean that it hasn't worked or that you are the 'wrong' shape, as it's purely a reflection of how difficult the fitting process is. It's the equivalent of walking into a shoe shop not knowing your shoe size and trying on every shoe in order to find the best fit. You want the pessary to push up against your pelvic organs in order to correct their position so that the muscles can tighten there, while at the same time feeling comfortable enough that you can forget about it once it's in.

Where and what sort of prolapse we have will also dictate the type and size of the pessary that is most suitable. You shouldn't have to figure this out on your own. If you are worried about prolapse then you must visit your GP, gynaecologist or women's health physiotherapist. They will help you to map out what's going on and recommend the best size and shape of pessary for you or give you information on where and how to get one fitted. Often it is trial and error, but this is not something you need to do on your own nor feel embarrassed to discuss with any medical professional. It is just another type of cast for an injured body part. You wouldn't dream of telling an A&E doctor what size, material and type of cast you would like on your broken arm and your vagina is no different.

I'll always recall watching in horror an episode of *Call the Midwife*, a brilliant quintessentially British drama set in the late 50s, where an older mother was putting up with the discomfort of a pelvic organ prolapse and inserting a potato inside herself to hold everything in place (yes, a potato!). When her secret was outed there was no shame, just many tears of empathy and heaps of support. She was seen by a gynaecologist in the very same episode and we got to observe a kind consultation between herself and the doctor about her treatment options. No more potatoes, no more embarrassment, no more accidents.

Three Types of Pessary

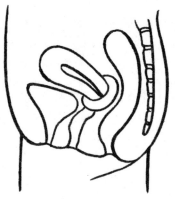

Ring

Gelhorn

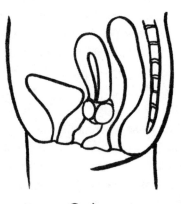

Cube

My story continued

I wore a pessary through my second pregnancy and often use this detail to reassure women that they're not only safe, but can also help prevent injury. From the fifth month of pregnancy I was feeling pretty heavy down there, my labia were swollen and riddled with varicose veins, and the end-of-day discomfort from my muscles straining to hold everything up was draining. These are all very normal feelings in pregnancy and especially after pre-existing birth trauma. I was feeling nervous about my brother's upcoming wedding where I inevitably would need to be on my feet and, worse, dance! While I was continuing to exercise every day, with the unsteadiness and pain at the front of my pelvis, coupled with my darling Coco growing at a rate that I couldn't keep up with, I knew this would be an activity much too difficult for my already challenged pelvic floor, so I went back to see Demetri. He knows me well and knows that resting with my feet up to offload the pelvic floor was an unrealistic option given my job as a physiotherapist, my love of exercise and the fact that I am a mother, so he fitted me for a ring pessary which gave my body the support it was lacking. I managed to dance at my brother's wedding, taking rests every few songs, thankfully only because I needed to catch my breath and not because of pelvic floor discomfort. I kept the pessary in right up until I started maternity leave, when I could rest more, and remained free of prolapse symptoms right up to the very end.

And so pessaries are not just for old ladies and are definitely not for forever. That said, you are not a failure if you need one long term. In fact, there are many times when wearing a long-term pessary is a good option and some injuries warrant this, for example, when the trauma has been significant, when there has been a nerve injury or following several gynaecological surgeries. These all impact on the success of pelvic floor strengthening.

Protecting and stabilising are the precursors to rehabilitating, but continue with what you have learnt in these two phases as we progress to rehabilitate. Your greatest success will come when you are protected, stable and stronger.

Rehabilitate

If you have a pelvic organ prolapse you need to exercise and strengthen the overloaded muscles. If they were left alone they would become weaker and inevitably the descent of the pelvic organs would worsen. I challenge the recommendation that I've heard recklessly given to mothers presenting with prolapse to 'rest and not do anything'. If we do nothing how can we expect things to change? Especially as we still have a baby and maybe even older children to care for, a life to lead, a body to feel comfortable in and a sex life to resume. While I recognise rest, or rather protection, is essential, it is only one part of the healing process. Pelvic floor exercises are the front line treatment for prolapse, and should be recommended and taught to everyone in the first instance.

As with any muscle injury you need to restore the muscle as a whole. Part of the muscle is likely injured and weakened, while another is likely to be compensating for this. So, confusingly, the pelvic floor can be both lax and weak and short and tight! In the presence of pelvic organ prolapse, release work can be the piece of the rehabilitation puzzle that is missing, so please don't skip task 3 (page 55) thinking there's no way that you're too tight down there! Often with prolapse women can accidentally overwork the pelvic floor in an attempt to stabilise their bodies and protect them from discomfort, but what is actually needed is to fully relax so that they can fully strengthen. Clenching any muscle and keeping it tense is unlikely to provide us with the function we need.

When we rebuild we go step by step in order to prevent aggravating our symptoms, progressing only once we have achieved the strength needed, not because of the passing of time. It may take longer for you to work through this task than your friend or neighbour. That's OK. You may need more strength than her, have a different injury to her or just have a different vagina to hers! It's all normal. When you apply this progressive loading theory, you will grow stronger, so let's get started!

TASK 9 RAISING THE FLOOR

Remember your vaginal elevator, with its closing doors and lifting mechanism? (If you don't, see page 60–1.) That's exactly what you're going to do here, but under greater load and pressure to build even further strength.

Start with step 1 every day to teach the muscles where you want them to be and progress through the steps only when you can feel everything lifting and can perform them with ease. There's no time frame and it's not a race. It will take at least three months to strengthen a muscle and even longer if there has been an injury, so keep going until you feel strong enough.

KIT YOU WILL NEED: Soft Pilates ball, roughly 10cm in diameter and made of soft rubber. These are perfect for squeezing between your legs and are the perfect accessory for these exercises and many more to follow. They're also good for between your knees while you're working to keep your posture.

Where you see the phrase 'close and lift your pelvic floor,' perform your best pelvic floor elevator contraction, closing the doors and lifting the layers from the outside of your body to the inside (see pages 60–1). You can isolate each passageway in turn and alternate between them with each repetition or consider the pelvic floor as a whole. Aim to hold your best contraction in each exercise and add the movement on top. If you can't do both then you're not yet ready for this task, but keep going with task 4 or 5 (pages 58–67) and you will be ready soon.

Once you've learnt the exercise you can add in your outbreath and use the upward movement of the diaphragm to help your pelvic floor lift. How? Whenever you 'close and lift your pelvic floor' do it on your exhale. As you're holding, breathe normally with shallow breaths. As you release, breathe in.

STEP 1 – WORKING WITHOUT GRAVITY

Bridge: Lying on your back with your knees bent and feet flat on the floor, squeeze the ball between your knees and lift your hips up in the air. Ensure your pelvis is higher than your ribcage – imagine and maybe even sense your pelvic organs moving upwards. Hold this position and *close and lift your pelvic floor*. Hold this for as long as possible – up to 10 seconds. Relax your pelvic floor then lower your bottom. Repeat x10.

Once you can do this you are ready for the through-range version. *Close and lift your pelvic floor* as you squeeze the ball and lift your hips up, breathing out at the same time, so that when your hips are high you have reached the top of your pelvic floor contraction. Hold for 5 seconds then slowly lower your hips down, simultaneously releasing with control your pelvic floor as your bottom lowers. Repeat for 2-4 minutes or until you start to tire.

Heel squeeze: On your tummy with your legs bent like a frog, hold the ball between your heels. Squeeze the ball and then *close and lift your pelvic floor*. Hold this for as long as possible, up to 10 seconds. Relax your pelvic floor and release the squeeze. Repeat x10.

When you can, move on to the through-range version. Start with squeezing the ball between your heels, then bend your legs up and into the frog-legged position as you *close and lift your pelvic floor*. Hold at the top for 5 seconds, then relax your pelvic floor, release the squeeze and lower your legs all together. Repeat for 2-4 minutes or until you start to tire.

Supine overhead arms: Lying with your legs straight and the ball between your feet, squeeze the ball and then *close and lift your pelvic floor*. Hold this for as long as possible, up to 10 seconds. Relax your pelvic floor and release the squeeze. Repeat x10.

Move to the through-range version once you can do 10 seconds x10. Squeeze the ball, *close and lift your pelvic floor,* take your arms over head and hold for 5 seconds. Then return your arms, and release your pelvic floor and the ball squeeze. Repeat for 2-4 minutes or until you start to tire.

STEP 2 – WORKING ACROSS GRAVITY

Side-lying lower leg lift: Lie on your side with your top knee bent and resting on the floor in front of you, and your bottom leg reaching straight down. Keep your body long and try not to sink into the mat as you lift this bottom leg up towards the sky. Hold it here as you *close and lift your pelvic floor* contraction and hold until you tire, up to 10 seconds. Relax your leg then repeat x10.

Once you can do 10-second holds x10 you are ready for the through-range version. From the same position *close and lift your pelvic floor* as you lift your lower leg to the sky, release your pelvic floor as your leg lowers. Repeat for 2 minutes and then change sides.

Box ball squeeze: On your hands and knees, find the four curves of your spine and hold them in neutral. Squeeze a ball between your knees and *close and lift your pelvic floor*. Hold for 10 seconds, then relax your pelvic floor and release the squeeze. Repeat x10.

When you can do 10 seconds x10, progress to the through-range version. Squeeze the ball and *close and lift your pelvic floor* as you raise one arm off the floor and reach it out in front of you. Hold for 5 seconds, then release your squeeze and pelvic floor contraction as you return your arm. Alternate sides. Repeat for 2-4 minutes or until you start to tire.

High kneeling ball squeeze: In a high kneeling position, grow as tall as you can, showing off your necklace to the room. Squeeze the ball between your heels while you *close and lift your pelvic floor*. Hold for up to 10 seconds, then relax and release. Repeat x10.

When you can do 10 seconds x10, add some movement. Start with your bottom on your heels. As you *close and lift your pelvic floor* squeeze your heels together and lift your bottom up from your heels, so that you are now in a high kneeling position. Hold for 5 seconds, then release the squeeze and your pelvic floor contraction as you lower your bottom back down.

STEP 3 – WORKING AGAINST GRAVITY

Seated ball squeeze: Seated on a chair, squeeze a ball between your knees and press your palms together. Hold this position and *close and lift your pelvic floor*. Hold this for up to 10 seconds. Relax your pelvic floor and release the ball squeeze. Repeat x10.

Once you can do 10 second holds x10 you are ready for the through-range version. Start seated on the chair, squeeze a ball between your knees and press your palms together. *Close and lift your pelvic floor* as you stand up. Hold for 5 seconds, then slowly lower your bottom back down to sitting while simultaneously releasing your pelvic floor contraction and the ball squeeze. Keep the ball squeezed until you are fully seated. Repeat for 2-4 minutes or until you start to tire.

Split squat knee hover: From kneeling step one leg forwards and ensure there is a 90-degree bend in each knee. Lengthen your spine as much as you can and find your neutral pelvis position. *Close and lift your pelvic floor* and hold for as long as you can, up to 10 seconds. Release, relax, then on each side repeat x5.

When you can do a total of 10 seconds x10, start in the same position, but as you *close and lift your pelvic floor* , breathe out and press down through your back foot to hover your knees just a few inches off the floor. Maintain your pelvic floor contraction and hold for 5 seconds, then return to the floor, relaxing your pelvic floor. On each side repeat x10.

Weighted ball squeeze between knees: Adding weights with your pelvic floor contraction is the last step. Start by standing and find the four curves of your spine and your best posture by allowing your head to float skyward as though it is a helium balloon. Just hold the weight in your hands at your sides (2-4kg is plenty to start with) and squeeze the ball between your knees while you *close and lift your pelvic floor*. Hold for 10 seconds, then relax and release the pelvic floor, and reset. Repeat x10.

When you can do 10 seconds x10 incorporate movement as well. Add a lift of the weight when you *close and lift your pelvic floor*, hold for 5 seconds, and release your pelvic floor as you lower the weight. This could be a bicep curl, overhead arms or side raises. Mix them up to get through 2-4 minutes of work, synchronising your outbreath with every lift of the weights and simultaneous pelvic floor contraction.

It's important to remember pelvic organ prolapse is an injury. You can't expect the muscles to perform perfectly at first, nor will you be able to do these exercises while on the bus, driving or feeding your baby. This is healing and rebuilding, and I encourage you to take time and embrace the exercises needed to recover fully.

This is by no means an exhaustive list of exercises and you can include any that will help you to reach your goal. Decide what that is and then let's break it down. For example, if your goal is to carry your baby in their sling for 20 minutes, you could use this set of exercises:

STEP 1

Standing pelvic floor exercises while breathing and squeezing a ball between your knees for 10 seconds x10.

Progress: Add in overhead arms with your exhale. Repeat for at least 2-4 minutes.

STEP 2

Add a weight to the above exercise, either holding that weight in your baby's sling or just in your hands. Close and lift your pelvic floor and squeeze a ball for 10 seconds x10.

Progress: Raise the weight, or just your arms if the weight is in the sling, overhead. As you squeeze the ball between your knees exhale, and close and lift your pelvic floor. Release as your arms come down. Repeat for at least 2-4 minutes.

STEP 3

Add a movement to the weighted exercise. As you close and lift your pelvic floor, breathe out and lift your arms overhead, simultaneously lifting one leg. Lower everything together and then repeat with the opposite leg. Continue for 2-4 minutes.

To achieve your goal, break it down and practise regularly to grow stronger.

Surgery for pelvic organ prolapse

Some women with prolapse may be asked to consider surgical repair undertaken by a gynaecological surgeon. It is another option if for any reason you are unable to rehabilitate fully, or the severity, longevity or impact of your pelvic organ prolapse has been too great, but you may be reading this needing the reassurance that there is something else. You may well have heard, and consequently become terrified of, vaginal surgery whereby mesh has been routinely used to support a prolapsed uterus. This 'engineering' has been getting a lot of bad press recently and rightly so. Although it has been successful in reducing prolapse symptoms and was the gold standard surgery for pelvic organ prolapse for years, it has been found that over time the mesh can work its way free and into a woman's bladder, bowel or vagina, causing considerable pain and discomfort. However, according to the National Institute for Clinical Excellence (NICE), this type of surgery is no longer recommended due to its 'serious but well-recognised safety concerns'. Other, safer, surgical options still exist, such as an anterior or posterior wall repair, which involves cutting the muscles and re-stitching them closer together, or, in some cases, and providing you have finished having your family, a partial hysterectomy. Both of these cannot be taken lightly and are serious operations followed by lengthy recovery periods.

I strongly believe that the pelvic joints and supporting musculature need to be working well to have a good outcome from prolapse surgery. Before you even consider this major step, 'pre-hab' is essential to ensure your entire pelvic ring and its muscles are as strong as they can be. Of course, you need to address any compounding factors such as poor posture, pelvic pain and DRAM before you take drastic measures to surgically 'fix' just one part. The women I see with prolapse have an element of all of these symptoms and their whole body needs rehabilitating to get the best outcome with or without surgery. Treating just one part instead of the whole is, in my view, the unfortunate reason that prolapse repair surgery doesn't have great success rates. Operative solutions are really only the best option for a minority of women and this should be discussed carefully with a gynaecologist.

Real-life story

Luciana is a mum of two and a prolapse survivor

I first learned I was pregnant on 1 January 2016. My husband and I had been trying for over a year, so this came as the most wonderful surprise and the absolute best way to start the new year. I was living in Singapore at the time and felt that I was in the best hands possible, and that my doctor would do whatever it took to ensure that both me and my baby were healthy. In hindsight though, I don't recall my doctor mentioning anything related to the pelvic floor, the potential issues that could arise during birth or what I needed to know once the baby arrived.

In what was my last prenatal check-up (week 39), my doctor told me I needed to be induced. I was very scared about the potential risks for my baby if he was stuck in the birth canal for too long. However, that wasn't the case as the day came around and my pushes were so forceful that he was born in just 12 minutes, but I sustained a bad tear and also, I later found out, an injury to the muscles inside my birth canal.

At around six weeks after his birth I was out for a walk and suddenly I felt something wasn't right, like a tampon out of place, and I hurried back home to check what was going on. To be honest I didn't even know what I was seeing in the mirror… was my vagina swollen? I rang my doctor and requested an urgent appointment. When she examined me, she said in the most matter-of-fact way, 'Oh yes... you have a prolapse of the bladder. I did notice it during your first check-up, but I thought it would be gone by now.'

At that moment I felt my world come to a screeching halt. I fell into a rabbit hole, constantly searching about the condition, looking for 'magical cures' and healing therapies. I entered the most terrible depression where I re-lived every second of my birth, hated my body and felt jealous of every woman out there that didn't have this condition. Desperate to find someone who could help, I joined a Facebook group for women with prolapse and became friends with two other women that lived nearby. We formed a sort of support group and talked about issues that only we could understand. We worked with the same physio towards our own individual rehabilitation plans and met up every Tuesday night for a pelvic floor Pilates class that she designed especially for us. Aside from working on our pelvic floors and strengthening our bodies, these sessions turned into our safe space and in a way were therapeutic.

As time went on, I began feeling stronger both physically and emotionally, and my life slowly regained the sense of normality I thought had been taken away from me after the birth of my son. I began to move in ways that at one point had seemed completely impossible and my mindset shifted from being defined by my prolapse, to seeing it as something I needed to manage. Almost three years after my journey began, I became pregnant with my second baby; this was perhaps my biggest leap of faith ever! Luckily, I was in the hands of a midwife who knew about the OASI (obstetric anal sphincter injuries) protocol and with her help I was able to birth my baby without any further damage to my pelvic floor.

I know that my pelvic floor will be something I will probably always need to be mindful of, but I am living my life and that is all I ultimately hoped to do!

When to ask for help:

- You notice a bulge, heaviness or something moving into your vagina. This could be a natural stretch of your vaginal wall following pregnancy and birth that will resolve over time or it may be a sign of pelvic organ prolapse.

- You have ongoing constipation, a chronic cough or extreme vomiting (as a result of future pregnancies or otherwise). Such vigorous and continued straining can weaken your pelvic floor and increase your risk of pelvic organ prolapse.

- You suspect you may have or have been previously diagnosed with a prolapse and you are breastfeeding. Oestrogen levels drop significantly following pregnancy and they may stay low while you are breastfeeding. As the pelvic floor and the muscles of our bladder contain oestrogen receptors, this drop in oestrogen levels after pregnancy can contribute to laxity and prolapse symptoms.

What to ask for:

- A referral to a women's health physiotherapist for advice and prescriptive pelvic floor exercises. This is the first line of treatment for pelvic organ prolapse.

- A referral to a gynaecologist for the fitting of a pessary to act as an internal support during your post-birth recovery.

- Laxatives, stool softeners or dietary advice for constipation to tackle this common, easy-to-ignore but problematic post-pregnancy symptom.

- Oestrogen creams and pessaries can be prescribed by your doctor to help with the healing of prolapse while breastfeeding. These are applied or inserted into your vagina to instantly help with muscle tone and the dryness that can come with having lower oestrogen levels while feeding.

What's important

- Pelvic organ prolapse can be thought of as simple physics – the load is more than the capacity of the muscles. Raise the capacity and you can handle the load. Your exercise intensity should be progressive to meet the challenges of your lifestyle and goals. We cannot stay at the same level or else we stay at the same capacity.

- Rehabilitation of a pelvic organ prolapse is both an inside and an outside job that needs to address pelvic floor strength alongside pelvic posture and abdominal wall healing.

- Use pessaries and modify your activities to *support* your rehabilitation, not replace it. This should be done in conjunction with your GP, gynaecologist or a women's health physiotherapist.

- Pelvic floor exercises are individual and specific to each of us – what we feel, our life's challenges and our goals. Your optimal pelvic floor exercises may not be the same as anyone else's. Tailor-make your own programme from my selection of exercises and progress when you have grown stronger, rather than doing them for a certain period of time. Progression is your key to long-term success.

7. Pelvic pain: Re-centring the keystone to strength

Keystone (noun):
1 *The middle piece that holds all other pieces in position.*
2 *The most important part in the plan or idea, on which everything else depends.*
3 *Something on which associated things depend upon for support.*

While we are looking more closely at the bones of our pelvis, the ligaments that connect them and its muscular walls, we cannot ignore the memories and experiences that are connected to this part of us. It truly is our centre and re-addressing its balance can unlock – or rather lock in – other pieces of our physical and emotional recovery. Its position and ability to change position can dictate our posture, pain and ease of movement. But it's also so much more than this. Our pelvis houses life, the organs which determine our sex and our sexual pleasure, and it is connected to our every breath. Many tiny movements pass through our pelvis each day and when we consider its many roles anything less than perfect just won't do. Our pelvis must provide us with a stable base from which to move and a secure door frame for our door – the pelvic floor. So let's take a look together and figure out what's up with yours.

The three bones of our pelvis slot together with reciprocal grooves like that of a jigsaw puzzle. Remember the two C-curved ilia connected at the front and at the back, at the base of our spine? Just like that last wedge-shaped stone at the top of an archway, our sacrum acts as a keystone for the ilia to snuggle up against and depend upon. Our pelvis is stable and strong just like that stone archway, but any change in position of the stones or bones compromises this stability, which can result in pain and problems.

Our pelvic floor muscles line our pelvis and so provide even greater stability by compressing the joints, drawing the bones together from the inside. This is like having a strong door in the archway to support your stone structure. Then there are the muscles on the outside of our pelvis, which provide even further support, much like the walls butting up against the archway do. Muscular injury, weakness and deconditioning from reduced exercise can compromise the support and stability our muscular system provides.

When we're pregnant it is natural for the joints between the bones of our pelvis to move more than normal as pregnancy hormones and weight gain make our ligaments and muscles stretch. At full-term pregnancy the joints of our pelvis can move apart even further as our baby's head becomes engaged and further still if we go into labour and we give birth vaginally. Our keystone moves out of its locked position to allow our ilia to move apart and our pelvis to 'open'. Our pelvic floor muscles stretch to allow our baby to descend and birth, impacting their ability to provide their normal internal stability and support. The change in our pelvis position can also make it harder for the muscles on the outside to provide strength as their start and end points have changed. The result? Pelvic pain that doesn't always resolve following pregnancy and birth, incontinence in late-stage pregnancy that can remain a problem years later and tummy muscles 'refusing' to snap back as they don't have the bony support or scaffolding to do so. These are not demonstrations of 'normal' pregnancy and post-natal complaints, but a result of the complexity of our muscle and skeletal systems and why addressing your back pain is crucial to keeping your knickers dry.

Another way of thinking about the relationship between our muscles and our skeletal system is to consider the structure of a tent. One of my first experiences of camping was at Glastonbury 2007. Needless to say the tent preparations were given little consideration until the rain came down. To pitch a tent you need to first put the poles together securely, then position the poles in their correct and interlocking places, just like the bones of our pelvis. Then there's the waterproof canvas to go over the poles that act as our walls, roof and floor, as do our core muscles. But this won't keep us warm and dry.

It turned out that while our tent looked good, it was up and similar to the picture on the label, we hadn't appreciated the value of guide ropes and tent pegs. Surely they were accessories and 'nice to haves'? And so after a long night's partying we came back to a flat pack version of what we had erected hours before. The missing guide ropes and pegs were just as, if not more, important than the main event.

Our multi-layered bodies are the same as that ill-fated Glastonbury tent. A skewed pelvis or curve in our back that is too big or two small will not support the canvas under which we need to shelter. The canvas, our muscular walls, pelvic floor and diaphragmatic roof, are the important parts, the tent as we know it, but without the bony tent poles the canvas on its own will never make a good tent. Just like our bodies, a tent with secure poles and a well-fitting canvas can function, but will it weather the storm? As the wind blows and pregnancy changes the shape of our poles and canvas we need the guide ropes and tent pegs to hold us firm. The bigger muscles of our thighs, back, bottom and bellies become our anchors and not our 'nice to haves'. These muscle systems act like tent pegs to support our bony pelvis and pelvic floor through pregnancy, birth and our recovery thereafter. Together these multiple layers make us strong and stable, warm and dry.

I often hear mums say, 'My pelvis is wonky.' It can happen and does often. With a vaginal delivery the joints of the pelvis will reach their maximum stretch, almost double the normal gap between our bones, as our baby enters the birth canal and is born. In most cases the joints will return to near their natural resting position in the weeks following birth, but not always. In some cases the pelvis remains 'open'. You may be aware of this and sense instability, pain or just feel different in your pelvic area. Women often tell me they can't trust their movements or their pelvic floor, as though it's out of their control, or they feel their pelvis could break in half, like a wishbone, at any moment. Sometimes they are totally unaware that their pelvis has changed position at all, but painfully conscious that their pelvic floor and tummy are not as strong as they were before. We can't take the changes our pelvis makes to accommodate life for granted or assume that our pre-pregnancy pelvis form and force will be automatically restored.

When things go awry the first feature is often pain. Regardless of pregnancy, both women and men, young and old can experience pelvic pain and pain is a great indicator that all is not well. Pelvic pain may manifest at the front of your pelvis, underneath, at the back on one or both sides, in your bottom, hips or lower back. But impairments can be present even when pain isn't. Maybe you don't have pain, but you leak urine, poo or wind, or experience pelvic organ prolapse or another impaired function of your nether regions. This can be just as much down to the pelvic ring as the pelvic floor muscles themselves.

Pubic symphysis pain

The front bones of our pelvis meet at our pubic mound, a lovely term for that hard bony part where our pubic hair sprouts from, but the join between them can become painful and inflamed when it is too open or too pinched. Some women also notice a popping sound or sensation and may even feel movement here, which can be excruciatingly painful or, the opposite, completely numb. This is symphysis pubis dysfunction, also known as SPD, and risk factors for SPD include:

- Standing in lordotic posture, the Kardashian derriere from chapter 2, which can open up a gap in the joint at the front.
- Metabolic (calcium) and hormonal (relaxin and progesterone) changes that come with pregnancy and stretch the ligaments.
- Weakness of the supporting muscles as a result of pregnancy or lack of exercise.
- Trauma to the bones of the pelvis from falling, direct blows or traffic accidents.
- Significant weight gain.
- A very long, drawn-out second stage of labour that sustains the stretch on the pelvic joints or, the opposite, one that is super-fast and doesn't give the pelvis time to open slowly.
- Shoulder dystocia, where the baby's head is born, but there is a delay in delivering their shoulders. Often a McRoberts manoeuvre is performed to birth the baby and doctors and midwives will push one or both of the

mother's legs forcefully up towards her chest to create greater space to birth the baby. This can stretch any of the joints of the pelvis far beyond where they would 'naturally' go.

Sacro-iliac pain

Also called pelvic girdle pain or PGP, this is typically pain in 'the back pockets of your jeans', right where the pelvis bones meet the spine at the sacrum. It can come with pain at the front joint too or in the joints higher up in the back. Risk factors for pain at the back of the pelvis include:

- Lop-sided pelvis – PGP is more prevalent when there is more strength and stability on one side compared to the other.
- Sway back or 'flat bottomed' posture (see page 36), which opens the joints at the back of the pelvis.
- Weight gain, especially that in pregnancy, because when the body is in sway posture the weight of the baby and swollen uterus sit right on top of these joints.
- Sudden increase in activity – undertaking a new sport, work or hobby.
- Forces that over-stretch the joints, such as falling, a traffic accident or even labour.
- Hormonal changes (namely progesterone and relaxin) stretching the ligaments.

After pain the second sign of an impairment in the pelvic ring is reduced muscle control, making certain activities more difficult. Pain and inflammation bog down the normal nerve messages to the muscles. Normal activation and function is replaced by guarding, spasm or these muscles being switched off altogether. This means, as well as pain and perhaps prolapse, we may feel weaker, have a low tolerance for exercise, experience fatigue and even wet ourselves. When there is a problem with any of the joints of the pelvic ring, typical movements which provoke such symptoms are:

- Weight-bearing – standing and loading these joints with your bodyweight and gravity.

- Walking, particularly fast walking, which demands greater movement at your pelvis.
- Standing from squatting, which tests the ability of your body to take the pelvis from a relatively open state to a more compressed state.
- Large single leg movements, such as getting out the car or bath and rolling over in bed.
- Lying on our backs – carrying a load straight across the sacro-iliac joints instead of your sitting bones.
- Standing up from sitting, which requires your keystone to rock forwards and lock into position. This can be painful when it is stuck.
- Opening your legs – stretching the front joint and compressing those at the back.

With stretching, strengthening and perhaps manual therapy with a physiotherapist you can restore your keystone's position and your posture. No matter how far down the post-natal road you are, please consider the role that your pregnancies and births play in the way your pelvis and subsequently your pelvic floor functions now. Prevention and even treatment can be as simple as protecting yourself from problematic activities, stabilising your keystone's most stable position to hold your 'arch', and strengthening your foundations and the muscles which cross the pelvis on the outside.

Protect

We know that lopsided movements, like carrying a toddler on one hip or crossing our legs, are the most likely drivers of pelvic pain. If pain arises when one side is moving more or less than the other, we need to take a look at where this can happen. When I sit at my desk I love to cross my right leg over my left and tuck my right foot around my left ankle, like some sort of leg pretzel! When I do this my whole right-side spirals inwards, opening my right pelvic joint at the back and closing the pubic joint at the front as I squeeze my legs together. To stop myself falling off the chair I have to rotate my left leg outwards, subconsciously working my left bottom and thigh muscles – making these work when my right side is relaxed. This asymmetrical pelvic position and muscle pull will create tension through my pelvic floor muscles and pelvic organs, make for a lazy tummy and back with an overcompensation in other areas.

Fortunately, as a physio I don't spend much time sitting, but when I do, I try to remember this and hold a ball between my knees to keep both inner thighs equally active or have a mini loop around the outside of my knees to keep both bottom muscles engaging. Better still, use both together and alternate between squeezing in and working the front and pressing outwards and working the back. If you have a desk job or spend lots of time in a car (not when you're driving obviously!) it's a good idea to employ this tactic too. I've also thought about other asymmetrical activities that might pop up in our lives and how to adjust for them.

Sleeping

Most of us prefer to sleep on one side more than the other and while side lying is the best position in pregnancy, after having a baby and throughout life, eight hours a night with a weight pressing down on one side while the other relaxes on top can take its toll. The goal when we're sleeping is to maintain the same neutral spine and 'best posture' when we're lying as when we're standing. Pillows are the perfect prop for this. One large pillow between our legs is often enough to keep our pelvis bones stacked on top of one another and to prevent our pelvis twisting forwards or backwards. I took this up in pregnancy and have never given it up. It is essential in pregnancy if you have or have ever had back or hip pain or just as a preventative measure. You can also double up and stop the pelvis moving up or down on one side with a small pillow at your waist. This keeps your spine straight instead of curving into the bed like a banana.

Desk set-up

More and more I hear of workspaces with two or more monitors to view. It's impossible to sit and face either monitor effectively and so we twist our body to see one or the other or both. Or perhaps you draw, use a mouse or write a lot – using one side of your body more than the other? Perhaps you're a dentist or surgeon and you have to contort your body so that you can use your dominant hand more efficiently? There are heaps of workspace tools and kit on the market to modify our desk set-up and workspace, but we can also adopt the ball between the knees or band around the thighs strategy to create equal loading or pressure at our base, even when our upper body activity cannot be equal.

If home is your workspace, you're a full-time mum or have a new-born baby to sit and feed, take heed of the desk set-up advice. This is your workspace. Consider where you spend most of your time and make it work best for you. We ideally want our bottom at the back of a chair and the whole length of our back supported, with both feet rested on the floor to stop us crossing our legs or wanting a foot stool. If you're shopping for a nursery chair, pay particular attention to the length of the seat pad. When you're sitting down measure the length of your thigh from behind your knee to where your bottom stops. This is the maximum length you want in a chair's seat pad. If this is too long for you, you'll not be able to get your bottom to the back and keep your spine long.

Driving

In a manual or automatic car our left leg gets a lot more rest than our right. If you spend a lot of time driving, then take a look at your leg position in the car. While we cannot change the asymmetric activity, we can ensure there is equal load or weight at the top of our legs under our sitting bones – at our pelvis. With our right leg out straight on the accelerator our right pelvis is likely to rotate backwards. Using a wedge underneath our bottom or just tilting our chair position so the bottom is higher than the knees can stop us excessively using this right pelvic joint over the left.

Standing in catwalk posture or 'propping up the bar'

Next time you're at a party, at the school gates, in a queue or at a work event take a look at how everyone is standing. Do they have both feet placed equally on the ground and do both knees have the same amount of bend in them? Unlikely! The natural, and least energy-consuming posture to take up is one hip out to the side, knee locked, weight in the heel and the other leg turned out, relaxed and carrying little load. However, I'm sure I don't need to point out what is happening up through the pelvis, low back, tummy and pelvic floor (very little if you're still wondering!). Everything is switched off. In this position we are hanging out, relying on our skeleton to hold us upright. Whenever I point this out to clients, they instantly correct themselves, take their feet hip width apart and stand up tall, everything engaged and switched on. This lasts 30 seconds maximum before they fall back into a much less effortful posture. So, let us compromise. If you work at a standing desk or counter, then you can always use the ball between your knees or band around the outside of your legs to maintain pelvis symmetry and stability, but in most social situations this would seem a little odd! Instead, move one foot forwards, as though you're going to take a step. When in this position, both legs are active front and back and one leg is not loaded more than the other. Or if you try a wider step than normal, with the toes turned out your bottom naturally fires up. If it doesn't (and you remember) squeeze your bottom muscles in this position for a 'free' activation exercise.

Baby feeding

Breast or bottle, it is likely you will tend to favour one side. Or perhaps you have to prop your baby up with a knee, simultaneously feed a toddler, or contort yourself into circus-style positions to feed in bed without waking up your partner and the small people who have also migrated into your bed! Even when you think it isn't, it's so worth setting up in the best feeding position before your baby latches on to breast or bottle. When your baby is bottle fed, often the mother's (or the father's) positioning is given less consideration. While you can manoeuvre a bottle more easily than a breast, you are still supporting the weight and optimal feeding position of your baby (or babies) and maintaining this for what often feels like hours. You will likely slouch forwards so that you can support your baby on your lap and hunch your shoulders to maintain their feeding position. Feeding pillows are definitely worth the investment and note that they are not just 'breast' feeding pillows. They lift your baby up to chest height so that you can keep a flat back and have one hand to hold breast or bottle and the other to comfort and caress your baby.

I didn't have a feeding pillow the first time around and thought I could make do with the cushions I had, which were never where I wanted them or the right shape. Second time around we had a few days on the neonatal intensive care unit. While being admitted here was scary, within just a few hours it was clear our Coco was OK, just very very hungry! Prophylactic antibiotics meant that we stayed in just to be sure and that Coco got what she needed. Every time I sat down to feed a wonderful nurse would whip out a feeding pillow and slip it under my baby, lifting her to the best position, then correct my posture with pillows for my back and arms so that I was relaxed and I could feed her comfortably. I had both my hands free to negotiate her latching on as the weight of her body was supported by the pillows. I could also rest both my shoulders back, sit upright without leaning to one side and relax. It was a true blessing to learn this and I kept it up at home.

You're going to be holding your baby, a breast and/or a bottle for hours and hours a day, so set up the space like you would your desk! Use pillows to support your posture and your baby. If you are tall one feeding pillow may not raise your baby enough and you may need a regular pillow underneath your feeding pillow to support them at the perfect height for you. Hold a ball or cushion between your knees to stop you from crossing your legs and try to change arms or sides at every feed. When you are relaxed and comfortable it is likely that your baby will be too.

Carrying toddlers and children on your hips

You probably can't avoid lifting and carrying little ones all the time, but you can hold them more efficiently and in a position less likely to cause you pain. Try having them front on or on your back with their legs wrapped around you like a koala hug, instead of all on the one side. You can also invest in a hip seat carrier – soft belts with inbuilt seats for toddlers so that you avoid jutting out your pelvis to create a ledge for them to perch on. This is also a good idea for your baby when they have head control and are wanting to be more upright and with you.

Maybe you feel these scenarios aren't relevant to you. Maybe you're already doing all of these things but still have pain. Sometimes we do what we think is right and what our body needs, and it feels worse afterwards. Like resting. Rest is a huge part of protecting yourself after pregnancy and birth. Our bodies need to heal and recover, but we need to give this some thought. Time spent resting is an opportunity to support and fix your pelvis in its best, most supported, locked position. If we hold it where it needs to be we will feel less discomfort when we change position, stand or move around. Here are some practical examples:

- Sun lounger position: Now relaxing on a sun lounger may not be an everyday occurrence, but how many of us have an L-shaped sofa and recline on it like a sun lounger? Or sit in bed with our legs out straight while reading a book? These positions tuck our bottom underneath us. This not only stretches the joints at the back of the pelvis, but also the back of the pelvic floor where it becomes slack and buckled. We are weight-bearing on our pelvic joints and not on our sitting bones, which were better built to carry this load. Instead, try lying on your tummy or your side (with cushions between your knees) to prop your pelvis (and its muscles) into a more optimal position. Sitting is OK and, of course, necessary at times, but ensure your back is upright and fully supported, and both of your feet can touch the floor in order to get your bodyweight right on top of your sitting bones.

- Bucket seats: A chair which is lower at the back than the front or that has a long seat depth will again make you rock backwards off your sitting bones and create a gap at the back of your pelvis. Look for a seat that you can get your bottom to the back of and that gives your back support. You should be able to rest your feet on the floor and your knees should be slightly lower than your bottom.

- Racing car position: And not just racing cars, but any car that is low to the ground where your bottom is lower than your knees. We just down-sized our car to a Mini and within a few weeks I could feel a discomfort in my lower back after driving. I had to adjust the seat to lift my bottom up and straighten the back rest so that I could sit on my sitting bones and not on my tail bone. Many cars now have the function to adjust your sitting posture, but if not play around with cushions to get your bottom above your knees and your weight on to your sitting bones while still being fully supported.

- Bath-tub: While soaking in the bath sounds tempting, this is just like lying in the sun lounger position. The heat from the water will also stretch your ligaments and muscles even further, which is exactly the opposite of what this rest, recover and protect phase is all about. If you have back or pelvic pain, or pelvic floor dysfunction, I recommend not taking baths. This position will stretch and put pressure on the back of the pelvis, its ligaments and pelvic floor, and you may notice your discomfort increase afterwards. Instead opt for showers and if heat feels like a comfort to you try using hot water bottles or warmed lavender bags. Set yourself up in a good spinal position, such as lying on your tummy or sitting upright, and then pop them over your pain where you need the relief.

- Baby changing: Baby changing tables are the nemesis of pelvic stability when you are tall or simply not the perfect height for which they were made. Leaning over a changing table will round your lower back, gapping the pelvic joints, buckling the tummy and pelvic floor – sub-optimal! Instead, try changing your baby while kneeling. This position tips your pelvis into a locked position and stacks all your vertebrae above, reducing the likelihood of pain in this position. Your pelvic floor sits in perfect tension, and your tummy and back muscles are active. Place your baby on your bed, chair or sofa, kneel on the floor and squeeze your heels together as you change them. You will hold your best posture and get a free workout at same time!

Correction of these every day movements can be all the protection our body needs. Sometimes it's not about doing more, but looking at what we're already doing and making this serve us better.

When I see new mums in pain I also ask them to consider pain relief as protection. Just resting is not always an option when you have a new baby to care for, but if you are in pain you are more likely to move differently and compensate in other ways you may not even be aware of. Where pain and swelling is present the very muscles we need to work cannot, so sorting out the pain is one of the very first steps in rebuilding our pelvic ring. Don't be afraid to discuss pain relief options with your doctor. Often pain relief is wrongly seen as a passive treatment 'masking' the problem. This is not the case if you do it in conjunction with other practices or as part of this progressive rebuilding plan.

Stabilise

If things are feeling stiff, tight and sore, or if you struggle to see changes in your posture, then there is likely to be tightness in your ligaments and muscles holding you back. Revisit task 2 (see page 39) to both relieve pain and support you in your best posture. If you are still struggling with pain, then I recommend visiting a physiotherapist as soon as possible in order to readdress your stability and alignment, and optimise your strength.

As well as protection and modifications to our home, movement and rest patterns, we can support our pelvic ring stability in many ways. While the ultimate stability comes from muscle strength, it's unlikely we can generate all the strength we need immediately, so at first we need to look at other ways to create this.

Pelvic stability belts: If you have had a traumatic birth, a history of pelvic pain or hypermobility syndrome (more on this on page 109), a pelvic stability belt is a great idea. Both the Baby Belly Pelvic Support Belt and Serola (and many more besides) provide external compression directly around your pelvic ring, bringing it together and providing a stable base from which to move. A pelvic stability belt should be worn for at least six weeks after the birth of your baby, alongside manual therapy and strengthening.

Core shorts: Just like a belt, these provide joint compression and can be easily worn under clothes. They are beneficial for stability in everyday movements, but also on return to sports and exercise after pregnancy and birth.

Pelvic taping: I often teach self-taping strategies as these are the best way of providing specific and tailored joint stability. You can stick the tape on right where you need it, which may be in a different place from day to day. Taping is as dynamic and changeable as your body. I use Rocktape and run two strips up either side of the spine from the sacrum up to the bra strap, then a third piece wrapping across the lower back from hip to hip.

Strengthening: You knew it was coming – the active part! When there is a problem with movement we need to reduce the amount of movement taking place. If you think of pregnancy and birth as events that move the body too much, we need to counter this with keeping things still, so the best strengthening exercises are those where you do a static hold. Anywhere we want to stabilise we should not move too much. Instead, hold it still, keep it steady, loading and strengthening it in the most stable position. It also makes sense to do things symmetrically and with both of your feet on the ground, instead of holding the weight of them in the air, what we call 'closed chain'. We need to achieve this before we can progress to through-range movement and single sided movements. While walking is often considered safe for early post-partum exercises, it is neither a static or closed chain exercise, and therefore can move you too much. We are often advised to avoid strengthening exercises for the first six weeks after pregnancy and birth, but that walking is OK. In my opinion the reverse is true. Stability comes not just through the passing of time, but also by strengthening our muscles to provide the support our body needs.

TASK 10 FIRST STEPS IN PELVIC STABILITY

KIT YOU WILL NEED: Just yourself, a floor/mat and a ball.

You can start these exercises from as soon as you feel ready to. They are my beginner exercises to relieve pain and lay down the foundations for strengthening. You need to put your pelvis in a position where it can be held, not twisted, shifted or bent. This happens automatically when you're lying on your tummy and when you are kneeling.

Whenever you see the phrase 'pelvic floor power', that's your cue to recruit all of the muscles from the outside, middle and deep layer (if you need a recap flick back to task 4 on page 58).

Prone heel squeeze: Lie face down with your legs straight, this naturally tips your pelvis forwards to lock in the joints at your back. Support your forehead on your hands. Start with your *pelvic floor power*, hold it and then add in a firm heel squeeze. Hold for 10 seconds x10, don't forget to breathe.

Heel squeeze in high kneeling: Just pressing your heels together will engage all the muscles at the back of your body, locking in not only your pelvic stability, but also good posture. In high kneeling, have your knees open but your heels touching. Grow as tall as you can as though your head is a balloon full of helium, floating up towards the ceiling. Start with your *pelvic floor power*, hold it and then press your heels firmly together. Hold for 10 seconds x10, and breathe as normal throughout.

Ball squeeze on your side: Lie on your side with your legs straight and feet directly in line with your shoulders so that there is length in your frame and you are in the best pelvic alignment while minimising the loading effect of gravity. Squeeze the ball between your feet and start your *pelvic floor power*. Hold for 10 seconds x10, and try not hold your breath.

Work on holding the positions for 10 seconds x10 on most days. In total that will make 5 minutes of work each day, which is perfect for addressing control and recruitment of your muscles.

Rehabilitate

Knowing how exactly to rehabilitate a painful, mobile or stiff pelvis can be a hard task, especially if this arises in pregnancy or after birth when you also have your baby's many needs to meet. Knowing that we have to complete this rehabilitation whenever pelvic stability has been compromised (as in pregnancy) is just as hard, especially when there is no pain to remind us! If you had a baby three months, three years or 13 years ago and have never completed specific pelvic stability rehabilitation, then this is a great time to

Muscular Slings

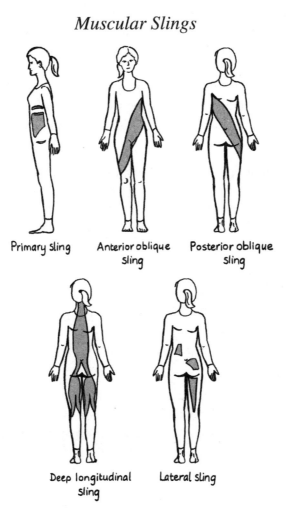

Primary sling   Anterior oblique sling   Posterior oblique sling

Deep longitudinal sling   Lateral sling

start. Whatever is occurring at your pelvic floor, back or tummy, or even if you're just working on prevention, work through these exercises and see how you perform. If they feel easy, that's brilliant, but if they feel hard stick with them, know that in fixing this you are fixing your whole system. Without a doubt unless we rehabilitate the pelvic ring then pelvic floor and tummy dysfunction is more likely.

Muscular slings are groups of powerful muscles which connect our upper and lower halves as well as our left- and right-hand sides. They work together to compress the joints of our pelvis into a stable position, hold us steady on one leg and reinforce our core strength. They are the supporting structures to the main event – our pelvic floor, pelvis and tummy. We will use them here to rebuild our pelvic ring strength, so it's a good idea to get to know what you're working with.

Primary sling: The pelvic floor, diaphragm, deep tummy and spinal muscles – this is active most of the time, including when we breathe, sit, move, rest or talk. Pregnancy and birth may compromise their action and we need to wake them up again.

Anterior oblique sling: The waist and opposite inner thigh, crossing through our pelvis and primary sling – this works to stabilise the front of our pelvis and therefore our pelvic floor and tummy. It's active when we step and walk – think about how we swing our arms, moving our opposite arm and leg forwards. A widening of our pelvis, pelvic floor or tummy muscles may make its action compromised.

Posterior oblique sling: The muscles from our shoulder blade at the back across to our opposite buttock over the back of our pelvis and primary sling – this closes and holds together the sacro-iliac joints at the back of our pelvis and works on the backwards part of our stride to pull our leg back behind us or climb up on a step.

Deep longitudinal sling: A straight line of muscles running along our spine, down to our bottom and back of our thigh – this gives us stability when we are on one leg and strength to straighten up our bodies after reaching to the ground, tying our shoelaces or picking up our babies. One side can work harder than the other and lead to imbalance and asymmetrical pain patterns.

Lateral sling: All of the buttock, back of the thigh and opposite waist – this gives stability to our pelvis when we're standing on one leg. It's essential for preventing catwalk hips or waddling when we're pregnant and keeps our pelvis steady on top of our legs as we walk.

TASK 11 REHABBING THE WHOLE PELVIC RING

KIT YOU WILL NEED: Soft Pilates ball to go between your knees. A cushion is OK, but to master these exercises it's worth investing in this piece of kit. You will also need a resistance band or cable strong enough to challenge your leg strength and a box, sofa or side table that can support your weight.

Where I say 'pelvic floor power', you need to recruit all of the muscles from the outside, middle and deep layer (if you need a recap flick back to task 4 – see page 58).

These exercises are progressive, meaning they get harder, which is why I've numbered them. Start at the first one and work through all those you feel able to do, one after the other, stopping when you struggle to perform the position for the required length of time. Work on all the exercises prior to this and including the one you're finding challenging. When you can do these drop the first exercise and pick up the next one in the sequence. Work on this until you can pick up the next exercise and drop the first and so on.

Always work on at least four exercises. If you can only do 1 or 1 and 2 to begin with, that's totally OK, but repeat them so that you're always doing at least four, although you can do more if you feel able to. You progress not because of time, but by achieving the next level. Work on these exercises three to five times a week to gain strength. Add on the next exercise only when you feel strong enough and have mastered those before it.

There are also two programmes here, A and B. One focuses on the front of the pelvic ring and one on the back. When you're in pain it's easy to work out which of these programmes you need to do. If you're not in pain try to work through all the levels of both and check you have equal strength through both the front and back of the pelvis. If not, work on the weaknesses.

PROGRAMME A: ANTERIOR (FRONT) PELVIC RING STRENGTH

Do this programme if you have: anterior pelvic floor dysfunction (urinary incontinence, bladder prolapse, sexual dysfunction), pubic pain, low tummy or inner thigh pain or strain, DRAM or low tummy muscle tone, or an increased arch in your lower back (lordosis).

1. Supine ball squeeze: Lying on your back with your legs straight, hold the ball between your knees. Add *pelvic floor power* as you take your arms over head. Exhale as your arms raise up, inhale as they lower. Make sure your body doesn't sway on the mat, keeping a neutral spine throughout, not allowing your back to lift away from the floor nor flatten into it. Repeat for 2 minutes.

2. Four point ball squeeze: On your hands and knees, ensure your thigh bones are vertical and elbows slightly unlocked. Find your neutral spine position, with a little curve in your lower back and maintain it throughout. Squeeze the ball between your thighs and without rocking from side to side raise alternate arms, reaching out in front of you. Using your *pelvic floor power* to help keep you steady, paying particular attention not to rock or lose shape when you change arms. Work continuously for 30 seconds, alternating your arms, then rest for 10 seconds. Repeat x4.

3. Hip twist open chain: Lie on your back with your knees bent and find your neutral spine, this means keeping a slight curve in your lower back and not flattening completely against the ground. Raise one leg and bend its knee. Keep your pelvis level by ensuring there is even weight under each side of your bottom and roll the lifted leg out to the side from the hip. Really focus on moving your leg without your pelvis or your lower back. Inhale as the leg rolls out, exhale and activate *pelvic floor power* as the leg rolls in. Continue for 1 minute then change sides. Repeat x2.

4. Table top ball squeeze: Your start position is the same as in exercise 3. But once you've lifted one leg, pause, *pelvic floor power* and then raise your other leg to join it, keeping your pelvic floor contracted so that your tummy doesn't pop out. Place the ball between your knees and squeeze it as you breathe, keeping tension through your tummy and your spine in neutral. Hold and breathe for 30 seconds, then rest for 10 seconds, lowering one leg down at a time, then repeat x4.

5. Side leg lifts: Lying on your side stretch out your entire body so that your feet are in line with your hips and shoulders, your tail is out and your neck is long. Keeping both your legs straight, first lift your top leg, breathe out, *pelvic floor power* and simultaneously lift the bottom leg. Lower both of your legs then repeat. Work for 1 minute on each side. Repeat x2.

6. Split kneeling hip hinge:

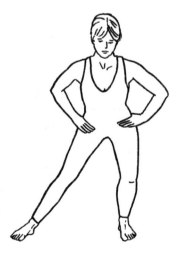

Start in a kneeling position with your shoulders over your hips and knees and take one leg straight out to the side. Bend forwards from your hips sticking your bottom out and bringing your body horizontal. then breathe out, *pelvic floor power* and thrust your hips forwards to bring your body back upright once more. Breathe out, relax and sit back again. Repeat for 1 minute then change sides. Repeat x2.

7. Standing skater:

Stand up and bend one leg taking your other straight leg out to the side and bending slightly forwards. Keeping both of your feet on the ground at all times press the foot of your straight leg down as firmly as you can into the floor as you drag it back in, with *pelvic floor power*, simultaneously straightening the supporting leg and coming back to standing. At the same time breathe out and activate your *pelvic floor power*. Breathe in and release as you return to your starting position. Repeat for 1 minute then change sides. Repeat x2.

8. Split side plank: Start sitting on your mat, take your legs straight out to one side and plant your bottom hand on the mat and keep the arm straight. Split your legs taking the top leg 6 inches or more in front of your bottom leg. Press through the outside of the underneath foot and the inside of your top foot and the palm of your hand, *pelvic floor power* and lift your hips up off the floor. Now you are in a side plank keep a straight line through your body with no bend in your hips. Hold and breathe with *pelvic floor power* for 30 seconds then change sides. Repeat x4.

9. Standing skater with resistance: This is just like exercise 7, but this time the straight leg has resistance around it. Attach one end of your resistance band to something firm that won't move and the other end to your straight leg. Pull your straight leg in as you stand up with the resistance of a band as you breathe out and start your *pelvic floor power*. Breathe in to release and return to your starting position. Unlike exercise 7, your straight leg now leaves the floor as you move in and out. Repeat for 1 minute on each side. Repeat x2.

10. Adductor side plank:

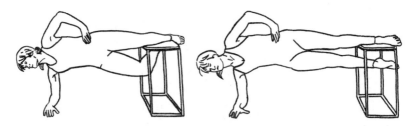

Start lying on your side with a box, side table or sofa level with your knees. Prop yourself up onto your bottom elbow and rest your top leg on your box. Ensure your top leg is bent and you are resting your inner thigh, knee and shin on your box. Next lift your bottom leg up off of the floor so your body weight is supported by your underneath arm and inner thigh of your top leg. Hold and breathe with *pelvic floor power* for 30 seconds on each side. Repeat x4. As you get stronger at this exercise move away from your box straightening out your top leg bit by bit until you can achieve this with a straight top leg with only its foot in contact with the box. The front of your pelvis is going to get heaps of pressure on it here to maximise stability. Sometimes this can be painful and pain is a sign you are not yet ready for this level. To help you get here try this exercise with your underneath leg on the floor to 'help-out' the top leg, carrying only as much load as you need to complete this exercise without pain.

PROGRAMME B: POSTERIOR (BACK) PELVIC RING STRENGTH

Do this programme if you have: pain at the back of your pelvis on one or both sides, posterior pelvic floor dysfunction (bowel or urinary incontinence, urgency, constipation or pelvic organ prolapse), flattened lower back, sway or flat-bottomed posture or tight hamstrings.

1. Isometric clam: Lie on your side and bend your knees. Ensure your shoulders, hips and heels are all in one line and your lower back is in a neutral curve before you lift both feet up off the floor. This should roll your top pelvis bone slightly in front of the one below. From here open your top knee while pressing your heels firmly together. Hold this with a *pelvic floor power* contraction for 1 minute then change sides. Repeat x2.

2. Kneeling hip hinge: Start in kneeling with your knees open and your heels pressing together firmly and your body leaned forward, shifting your bottom out behind you. Breathe out, turn on your *pelvic floor power* and push your hips up and though to a straight position stacking your shoulders over your hips and over your knees once more. Then release and sit back as you breathe in before repeating. Work on this continuously for 1 minute and rest for 10 seconds. Repeat x2.

3. Bridge from sofa: Your shoulders should be supported on your sofa, box or side table as you press through both of your feet to lift your hips up. In this position there should be a straight line from your shoulders through your hips to your knees. As you lift up breathe out and start your *pelvic floor power*, as you lower your bottom back down breathe in and release. Repeat x20 and rest for 10 seconds. Repeat x4.

4. Long lever kicks: On your hands and knees check that your thigh bones are vertical and maintain a very slight bend in your elbows. Keep your pelvis level and your spine in neutral as you straighten one leg out behind you, lifting it up in line with your hip. As it lifts, go for *pelvic floor power* and breathe out. Breathe in and release as it lowers. Try not to rock or sway and only move from your leg. Repeat x20 on the same side and then change sides. Repeat x4.

5. Supine plank: This can often be a hard one to master, but it is essential that your back strength here is equal to the front. Start sitting on your mat, your legs out straight and take your hands to the floor behind you. Keep your knees slightly unlocked as you lift your hips up in line with your shoulders and feet. Activate *pelvic floor power* here and breathe, hold for 30 seconds, then rest for 10 seconds. Repeat x 4.

6. Side plank with clam:

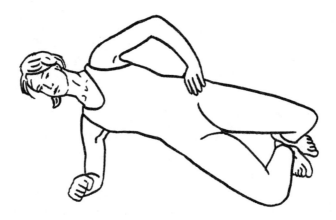

Lie on your side, bend your knees so that your feet stick out behind you and prop yourself up onto your elbow. Lift your bottom, waist and hip up off the floor so that you are weight-bearing on just your knees and your forearm. There should be a straight line down the front of your body from your elbow to your knee. Press your heels together with *pelvic floor power* and open your top leg. Breathe as you hold for 30 seconds if you can. Change sides – no rest. Repeat x4.

7. Bridge from sofa single leg: With your shoulders resting on a chair or sofa, lift your bottom up with both feet grounded. Once you are in position, engage *pelvic floor power to* keep your pelvis completely level as you lift one leg up off the floor to table top. Try not to let your bottom sink down as you hold for 5 seconds, then change sides holding again for 5 seconds before you lower your hips and release. Repeat x10.

8. Split kneeling leg lifts:

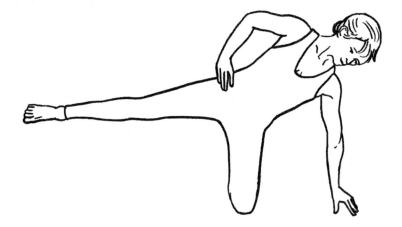

From kneeling, take one leg out to the side and bring your bottom hand down to the mat. Ensure there is a straight line through your body from this hand to your foot. Your weight-bearing thigh (the one with a bent knee) should be vertical and try to only have a little of your weight in your hand. As you breathe out start *pelvic floor power* and lift your straight leg up off the ground to hip height. Lower this leg, release, then repeat x15 before changing sides. Repeat x4.

9. Supine plank single leg: Just as exercise 5, but once your hips are up in supine plank keep your hips level as you transfer all the weight to one leg and raise the other to the sky. Activate *pelvic floor power* to help hold you steady here, breathe and hold for 30 seconds, then change sides. Repeat x 4.

10. Side plank single leg: Start in a side plank, weight bearing on just your feet and one hand and creating a straight line from this hand through your hip and between your feet. Keep your hips stacked and facing forwards and your spine straight as you *pelvic floor power* to hold it here. It may be enough to stay here, but if you can, raise your top leg to the sky so only one hand and one foot remain on the floor. Whichever position feels good, hold and breathe for 30 seconds, then change sides. Repeat x4.

When you find the correct stage in this programme for you, the challenge should feel real. Aim to complete at least 8 minutes' worth of work and feel like you have worked hard. As we are connected front and back you may need to work on both programmes simultaneously to regain your fullest strength.

These exercises use your own body weight to provide the resistance, but always consider your goals and what you need your body to achieve. The intensity of your rebuilding plan should match this. If you're a keen runner you will need to get to at least 10 because when we run at least three times our body weight will go down through one leg. Therefore, adding even more resistance to these exercises is the next step (if you need it!). This can look like adding a weight in your hand or a band around your legs or using speed and power to increase the load. For example, 10 becomes so much harder when you substitute a static hold for raising the bottom leg up and down, or dipping and raising your hips or even placing a weight around the underneath leg!

Real-life story

Alice, mum of two, learnt to put up with pain and wet pants

I've had a bad back for as long as I can remember, even before having my children. I can't say that I consider myself 'post-natal' seeing as my kids are now 10 and 7, but I can definitely say that things got worse after having them. I'd put my back pain down to bad posture and sitting at a desk for long hours, neither of which I thought I could change. After my pregnancies my pain shifted and settled into my bottom, and I didn't recognise my stomach anymore. It bulged out like I was still pregnant and I had to wear a pad in my knickers in-case a sneeze caught me off guard and I wet myself – all things I can't believe I put up with now as I write them down, but I thought this was normal because my mum friends had similar complaints.

I had no idea it was all related. The first time I had any idea was when the physio I was referred to for my back pain recommended a pelvic floor exam. I didn't know what I was doing when it came to pelvic floor exercises. Up until this point I hadn't thought to mention my bladder problems, but with her being so thorough in the search for what was causing my painful back I told her everything.

It turned out my weak tummy and pelvic floor were causing my bad posture, which was causing my back pain. I started a daily routine of strengthening exercises. Slowly my posture did change and my back pain eased. Now I know how to do pelvic floor exercises properly, I don't wet myself anymore. I do get the odd pain and this serves as a reminder to sit better and do my exercises!

When to ask for help:

- If pain is significant, stopping you from being able to live as you choose or sleep at night, then it is likely that you will need some hands-on treatment, such as massage or manipulation, from a physiotherapist, chiropractor or osteopath.

- If your pelvis feels unstable, like a wishing bone that could snap at any point.

- If you have been putting up with back pain, pelvic floor problems and tummy muscle weakness for too long and now have a very strong hunch that they are all related.

What to ask for:

- A referral to a physiotherapist, chiropractor or osteopath. After a thorough assessment they can provide or direct you to the best treatment to give you pain-free movement and direct your rehabilitation exercise programmes.

- A referral to a women's health physiotherapist if you suspect your pelvic floor to be implicated.

- Pain relief medication or acupuncture, which is another great tool to alleviate pelvic pain and is very effective during pregnancy and after. In some areas this is offered by physiotherapists both privately and on the NHS. There are also acupuncturists who specialise in women's health.

What's important

- Where there is pain or problems with our movement these are signs that our joints and muscles inside and out cannot function optimally. We need to address both together.

- The pelvic floor is the primary stabiliser of the pelvis. Optimal position and strength of the pelvic floor is step one to gaining pelvic ring stability.

- Task 2 (see page 39) may provide you with the pain relief and postural changes you need before mastering the tasks from this section.

- If you don't have time for rehab right now, you can improve your posture by improving your resting positions and working on pelvic ring closure:

  - Standing – take your legs wide or one foot in front of the other with your weight evenly distributed to keep your postural muscles active.

  - Sitting (and driving) – ensure your hips are higher than your knees to tip your pelvis forward. Move your bottom to the back of the seat to keep your spine supported. When you're sitting down hold a ball between your knees to stop yourself crossing your legs and keep your primary sling engaged.

  - High kneeling – use this posture for as many activities as you can as a free workout for your pelvis.

- Sleeping – aim for side-lying with a pillow between your knees to keep your pelvis aligned as you sleep.

- Strength is different for everybody. Progress your exercise and build your strength to suit your life, goals and challenges.

8. Tummy recovery: We've fixed the floor, but what about the walls?

No matter how long ago you were pregnant I'm sure you remember the shape your body took on to accommodate your growing baby: your rounded, swollen belly, all out front or all around, stretching the skin and muscles of your tummy unrecognisably; the widening of your pelvis and rib cage, unmistakeable in the discomfort of pre-pregnancy bras and trousers; and the protruding triangle tummy when you tried to sit up in bed, rising up like an alien as your muscles stretched apart and the effort of moving pushed your tummy up through your midline. Even though we can all see the changes to our body and to our tummy muscles in particular, we so often skip past their recovery. Not knowing what to do and being too tired, overwhelmed and busy to think about it, we are at a loss and simply hope that we will 'snap back'.

This chapter has very little to do with how we look, but is instead about how we feel. Without our tummy strength we have little 'core'. Without our core, our back, pelvis and pelvic floor will also struggle. When our tummy muscles are split down the middle we are much more likely to experience back pain, wet knickers and even pelvic organ prolapse. And it's not just physical symptoms that post-baby tummy changes gift us, but also damaging effects on our body confidence. The psychological wellbeing that comes with feeling our strongest and having a positive body image is often overlooked, not to mention the knock-on effect this has on our self-esteem in the workplace, at the playground and in the bedroom. Body confidence, or rather lack of it, can wreak havoc with our libido and can distract us from living as we want to. I love that the most common feedback from my 'strengthening for mums' classes is not focussed on aesthetics, but more along the lines of 'I'm so much stronger than I was before.' I always take that feeling as a combination of both body and mind.

Sadly, the information that is currently out there about tummy exercises after pregnancy and birth is confusing at best and often impossible, conflicting and down-right wrong. The mis-matched ideas that we hear about post-natal training dos and don'ts leave many of us doing nothing for fear of doing something wrong! To clear this up it is essential that we understand what is actually happening. My post-natal tummy is not the same as yours or anyone else's. Therefore our re-building exercises will not be the same either. Like any rebuilding programme it is a step-by-step process and when you do this no exercise is off limits. You can do everything eventually, so long as you build it up correctly. I'll show you how, but let's just take a look at what we're dealing with first.

The truth is 100% of women who carry a baby in their womb will have stretched and weakened abdominal muscles as a result. You can't get away from it. The normal pregnancy stretch of our tummy muscles begins in the first trimester as the womb multiplies in size. This continues more visibly in the second trimester and is unmistakeable in the third and so after every pregnancy every mother needs to reverse this overstretch and shorten their tummy muscles in order to prevent back pain, correct negative changes to posture and address pelvic floor problems. Regardless of how many babies you have had or the method by which you gave birth (Caesarean or vaginal delivery), it is the pregnancy itself that weakens our tummy muscles. Strengthening and rehabilitating our tummy muscles is not just a job for those who wish to return to exercise or previous levels of fitness, but crucial for all of us who wish to lead active lives, keep up with our children, be pain free and preferably do all this with dry knickers.

Remember the idea of our abdominal muscles making up the walls of our house and that they need stable foundations (a strong pelvis and back), a good (pelvic) floor and a weatherproof roof (our diaphragm) in order to be safe, stable and secure? Reminding ourselves that these elements are interlinked and rely on one another is really helpful here. Rebuilding often comes down to more than just one part. If you haven't already, jump back to the pelvic floor rehabilitation in this book and tick it off as part of your tummy rehab checklist. Pelvic floor strength may be the missing piece of your tummy puzzle (task 4 on page 58 is a compulsory exercise!).

What if I have a gap – are my muscles split down the middle?

As well as the natural tummy stretch that comes with pregnancy, most of us who carry a baby to full term will also notice a separation of the long muscles down the front of our tummy. This gap is necessary to provide space for our baby to grow, but should close again within eight weeks of giving birth (abdominal or otherwise). One in three mums will notice that their gap takes longer to close than this and this can be a result of diastasis recti abdominis muscle (DRAM), which literally translates as separated rectus abdominis muscle. It's commonly described as a split down the middle and mistakenly referred to as a mum-tum (eye roll, sigh).

DRAM is not a normal tummy stretch or consequence of being a mother, but an injury like any other tear in a muscle. It occurs when the two muscles stretch further apart than they can tolerate, so they split and separate, and this needs to be rehabilitated. The gap can be just around our belly button where the linea alba is naturally weaker or can extend above or below from here. In some cases the length of the gap can extend most of the way up the midline. The length of our gap is another measure of its severity – the longer the overstretch then the more rebuilding you have to do. A pregnancy DRAM is more common with increased age, number of babies and twins, but it is difficult, if not impossible, to prevent.

Pre-pregnancy, pregnant and post pregnancy abdominal muscles

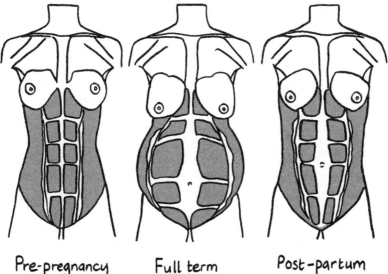

Pre-pregnancy abdominals

Full term pregnancy

Post-partum

In the majority of new mothers, both normal tummy stretch and DRAM naturally reduces in the first six to eight weeks post-birth. After this, recovery of strength will only come with rehabilitation. As I say, one third of us will have a DRAM beyond the natural six to eight-week recovery time and will need to focus on protecting, stabilising and rehabilitating to progress further.

DRAM is diagnosed when the gap between the left and right rectus muscles is more than 2.5cm. You may well see this written on your notes or referred to as IRD, your inter-recti distance (IRD), but I always take this with a pinch of salt. For those with a very slight frame a 1cm IRD can be hugely significant. Similarly, the classification of a 'moderate' DRAM at 3.5-4.5cm and a 'severe' one as more than 4.5cm can be misleading. Instead of the width of the gap dictating the severity, we need to look more closely at the depth. You may

Why tension matters, what it looks and feels like

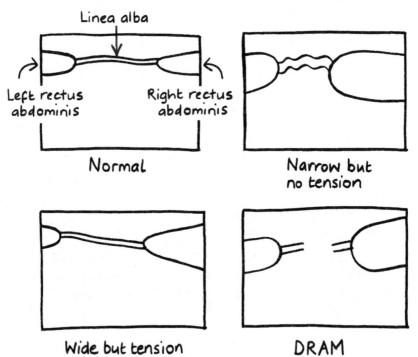

have a wide but shallow gap and recover better than if your gap is narrow yet deep. If your fingers sink deep into your linea alba (that connective tissue layer between your left and right side muscles) it is likely that this structure is very thin, weakened and may be torn. If there is resistance at the gap when you press your fingers down and they cannot sink deeply between the muscles then the linea alba is intact and although it may still be weak and thin, it can resist your probing fingers. This is what we call 'tension', a rigidity and tautness of the connective tissue between the left and right muscles. This is a good thing when it comes to our tummy muscle rehabilitation. I use depth *and* tension as an indicator of rehabilitation potential and recovery, rather than width alone.

TASK 12 TENSION TACTICS

KIT YOU WILL NEED: A ball to squeeze between your knees, a good pelvic floor contraction (recap with task 4 on page 58 if you need to check this) and an imagination!

To feel for tension place the fingers of your right hand firmly in the middle of your tummy between your belly button and your bikini line. Then place the fingers of your left hand at your midline between your belly button and your bra strap. You are not looking to feel a big bulging muscle, just a change in the firmness under your fingers and not necessarily under all of them at the same time. What you can feel is your linea alba, transversus abdominis corset muscle and the other abdominals which blend with it. You may be familiar with some of these cues from Pilates which targets the transversus abdominis, particularly in pre and post-natal Pilates. But remember this task is all about what is occurring at your midline. You may be great at 'Pilates' but if the cue you've always used isn't creating tension under your fingers then it's not the one to use right now. The midline should become taut like a trampoline and when you gently press into it with your fingers the depth should change from deep to shallow as you create tension. You may feel something underneath your fingers with all three of the following exercises, which is a good sign that this midline muscle is well connected. If you only feel tension with one or two of them then you can just work with these cues as they are the best ones for you. Sometimes you can't identify the tension building, but you can feel it release and that's good enough for me. It takes practise to sense the change in tissue tension accurately, but you just want to get to know how *your* body feels, so that you can track your progress.

Once you can feel the tension, try holding it while gently breathing for up to 10 seconds then releasing – you will notice the change in tension as you relax. Repeat this at least 10 times. It should begin to feel easier with every repetition (this may sound counterintuitive, but in theory these are muscles that don't get tired, so the more they're worked, the better they feel). Lying down is the easiest place to start in, but once you've mastered this move to high kneeling, then on all fours and lastly standing.

Pelvic floor elevator: When you engage all three layers of the pelvic floor, the deepest of your tummy muscles also engage and you can feel this as tension at your midline coming up just like an elevator, starting below your belly button, then at your belly button itself, then reaching just above it. Encourage this sequence by starting with the muscles at the outside of your pelvic floor. Imagine elevator doors at your vaginal opening and close them tightly. Then bring on the next layer of muscles inside your vagina as you pull that elevator up, and then the third layer, up by the neck of the womb, as you lift the imaginary elevator further inside. As you reach that third layer, or possibly from the second floor of your pelvic elevator, you may be able to feel this connection at your midline. What you can feel is the tension you need to build upon.

Baby hug: Try imagining you still have a baby inside your womb, filling up your tummy and stretching out your skin. Use your muscles to hug your baby, lifting them up and in towards your spine, closer inside you. Hug them gently and hold them there. If you struggle to do this with your muscles try it a few times with your hands. Lift that space belonging to your baby not that long ago up and in towards your spine. As you let go with your hands hold this position with your muscles.

The corset: Try to imagine how it would feel to wear a corset fastened with laces up the front. Start by tightening the bottom of your corset, down by your pubic bone. Pull on the strings, gradually moving upwards, tightening the corset, closing the two sides and at the same time feel your tummy draw together and up. Keep working on this tightening and pulling together, feeling all the way up your tummy to your belly button and maybe even higher if you can.

Tummy zipper: My favourite idea is imagining your tummy muscles as a (very) high waisted pair of jeans with its zipper being your linea alba running from your pubic bone to your ribcage. Use your muscles to close this zipper, ensuring you don't pinch your skin! Start at the bottom just as you would a zip, bringing the two sides and the two muscles together, working all the way up to your tummy button, closing and zipping left and right side together, up past your belly button all the way to your ribcage if you can.

Adductor squeeze: Your inner thighs make up the bottom half of your core strength, known as your anterior oblique sling, and together with your tummy muscles create a crisscross of strength straight through your midline. You can harness this strength to create the midline tension you're after. Start with your legs straight, a ball between your feet. Squeeze the ball and feel your tummy draw in and the tension build underneath your fingers. Try this with your knees bent and a ball between your knees. This works really well when combined with the above exercises.

Work on these every day until you can achieve 10 seconds x 6 in each of the following positions: lying with your legs straight, lying with your legs bent, kneeling and 4-point kneeling. You can alternate the cues or just work on one or two of these for the four minutes. This will set your tension, which is the foundation of all the exercises that follow.

Once you've learnt what tension feels like and how to create it the rest is simple… relatively. Creating tension across the gap is essential for rebuilding and the amount of tension we feel is the measure of our recovery potential. When there is tension and a shallow gap, regardless of its width, it means that you can transfer pressure across your midline when you move, lift, run or roll out of bed. Without it these activities and many more besides can be problematic. You may not have this tension all the time and it may take some work to find it, but this will be the basis of your tummy muscle recovery. During these tasks you may see your midline bulge outwards and dome, or you may leak or feel your back pain as your core cylinder struggles to cope, but this is the groundwork and foundation of everything else. If you can create tension in the middle then you can gradually increase the weight and pressure to get back to full strength.

To heal and rebuild from DRAM you need to select only the exercises which create your tension, ditching any which make the gap feel deeper. This way you will be specifically strengthening your midline where the injury is and not the rest of the abdominal wall. When I am rehabilitating those with a DRAM I spend 99% of the session with my fingers in their gap, feeling for tension and making sure that every exercise is creating strength exactly where it's needed most. If it's not creating tension, it's not the right exercise for you. While this might sound complicated you can easily become an expert in feeling for tension. With some practise you can get to know what it feels like to have tension at your midline or not. You're looking for an upward pressure against your fingers, a taut trampoline, your fingers being raised up, the gap not feeling so deep, a dense muscle or just a change. Get this and the rest will follow.

Lumps and bumps (AKA hernia)

For a few of us the stretch of our abdominal wall in pregnancy is so great that little tears appear in our linea alba. Loops of the bowel can push through these small holes and appear as one or several lumps. You may even be able to see your lunch moving inside your gut when you lie still! This is known as a hernia. Sometimes they are visible all the time and sometimes they only raise their heads when you lean backwards, cough or exercise.

The literature suggests that hernias occur in less than 0.1% of mums after pregnancy, but I'd suggest it's more like 10%. I increasingly find that when women come to see me for tummy rehab that doesn't seem to be getting anywhere they actually have a hernia, but most of the women don't know it's there. Perhaps this is why the documented occurrence is so low – not because they don't exist, but because we don't know they exist. In fact, this may be another frustratingly under-recognised, under-treated pregnancy-related injury.

If you suspect you may have a hernia the best place to start is with your doctor. They can refer you for a scan to diagnose the size, severity and type before helping you to decide what treatment path to go down. If your hernia is mild, surgery is often not required and you can work on rehabilitation to strengthen the area around it. Larger hernias, which risk your bowel getting trapped in the hole, will need a surgical repair. Sometimes this is a matter of stitching the two sides together, sometimes a surgical mesh is put in to close the hole. A surgeon will discuss this with you to decide which suits you the best.

Tummy muscle strengthening with a hernia means avoiding crunches, planking and similar exercises which increase the pressure inside your abdominal wall. Instead you work on strengthening the internal musculature, minimising the stretch on the rest of the midline and abdominal muscles. You are unlikely to fix a hernia with exercise alone as a hole is hole, but you can reduce the significance or impact of the hernia on your strength, tummy tension and shape. It's similar to doing up your coat. If the two sides of your zipper are not connected then the coat edges can move apart and your coat can open, but if you do the zipper up halfway then the top of your coat is also more secure, more together and less likely to move further apart. Likewise, if you zip up your tummy securely either side of the hole, then the hole becomes smaller and more together as a result.

My story continued

My second (large) baby left me with a hernia just above my belly button. I was obsessed with measuring it myself with the ultrasound machine in my clinic and was amazed to see it shrink in size as I grew stronger. After two years of healing and rebuilding it improved a lot, but I still had to be very careful with planks, press-ups and anything where I arched my back – yoga was off the table and I had to give up my beloved aerial acrobatics as it was definitely making it worse (think Anne from *The Greatest Showman*, but much, much less talented). I became frustrated as my recovery plateaued and despite my efforts there was still a 7mm tear at my bellybutton which my tummy could push through. My tummy felt like a bag with a hole in it. As much as I tried to fill it with strength, some would leak out. The bag was getting fuller all the time, but I couldn't get it full enough for what I liked to do – namely yoga in the air! I wasn't keen on a surgical repair as the recovery time is like that of a Caesarean section – eight weeks minimum with no lifting. This seemed impossible with a toddler. But after another injury (caused by a five-year-old jumping on to my tummy from the sofa) the hole got bigger and I hadn't much choice other than to have an operation. I underwent an umbilical repair at my local hospital. The hole was small enough for the surgeon to suture together, whereas larger holes may require mesh to be inserted to bridge the gap. It took six months for me to feel strong again and another three to get back to doing all the things that I enjoyed. I can now work and exercise without limitations. It wasn't an easy choice to make but as the surgeon put it: 'It is manageable until it's stopping you from doing the things you enjoy.'

Like most things, surgery is not a quick fix but a big step up the ladder and you still need to climb the rest of the way yourself. Once the wound heals the tension tactics from task 12 (see page 157) are a great place to start and from eight weeks you can follow the abdominal strengthening in task 15 (see page 173) just the same as anyone else. However, take it slow and steady, step by step, so that you don't re-open the hole and can continue to heal and rebuild.

Pregnancy and birth are 'hypermobile' conditions – ones where we get over-stretched – so our tummy healing and rebuilding is all about protecting ourselves from any further stretch and holding ourselves there. In some cases you may need to do this by wearing tape, belts or support braces, just as you would with any other injured muscle or bone. Then you can rebuild your strength bit by bit. Let's look at how.

Protect

Whether you gave birth last week or many years ago, you need to address everything that may be preventing your tummy muscles from healing – your posture, positioning, pain, the wrong type of exercise and your diet.

- Posture: I'm sure you already know how to flatten your tummy and I bet it starts by standing as tall as you can. If you stoop, slouch forward or sway backwards watch how your tummy pops forward. This is because the muscular corset we wear works best when we are in a good spinal posture, in neutral, with our rib cage over our pelvis, pelvis atop our hips, hips above our knees and our ankles directly below. Sway from this and you will lose your automatic corset and need to work a lot harder to maintain tummy tone and core strength. So whether you spend your days standing, sitting or moving around, take time to set up your best posture. Here are a few tips to keep your tummy engaged and to protect you from a 'passive pot belly'!
- Mix it up – whether you're working or resting, regularly swap between sitting, standing and perching on a high stool. This will prevent your muscles from tiring by being held in one position for too long.
- Step it out – try standing with one foot in front of the other, because it's much harder to slouch or sway. In this position you share your

bodyweight more evenly between each leg and both sides of your tummy will remain active.

- Sit strong – squeeze a ball between your knees when you sit to help maintain activity around your core and pelvic floor. This is an especially good use of time when you are sitting and feeding a baby. You can also try sitting on a balance cushion or gym ball to keep your core active (but not while feeding!).

- Grow tall – whether you're sitting or standing, try to grow tall from the crown of your head, as though there is a thread sprouting from your centre parting and you are being pulled up by this. Keep this in mind and practise it often. It will soon be a natural postural position for you.

- Open up – revisit the release work in task 2 (see page 39) to free up anything that's holding you back from achieving your best posture.

- Positioning: This is different from posture as it's all about aligning our bodies in the best position while we relax and rest. Sleeping, lying, sitting and feeding all require good form in order to aid our abdominal rehabilitation and prevent pain. We can rely on pillows, finding the best supportive chairs or just avoiding the ones which are not so good for us. We want to support our bodies in neutral – with the four natural curves of our spine, a dip in our waist and symmetry through our feet, hips and shoulders. When you're lying down try to lie on your side. Use a pillow between your knees to keep your pelvis bones stacked on top of one another and a smaller pillow underneath your waist to keep your waist from sinking into the bed. When you're sitting ensure that your bottom is higher than your feet so that you can keep a curve in your lower back and not buckle your abs. Sitting on a towel or cushion is best for this. Avoid sitting with your legs out straight, which again buckles the lower abs, and stretches the pelvis and lower back.

- Strip back your exercises: If you keep doing what you've always done, you'll get what you've always got. If you've been sticking to exercises that you thought helped but haven't, it's probably time to ditch them. Don't worry, I'm not suggesting taking exercise off the table altogether, but if you've decided to get stuck into healing yourself, let's look at everything, including stopping what is not serving you. Remember, in the post-natal period your body has moved too much, so your exercises should be focused on creating less movement. Every exercise must create a tension in the 'gap', a firmness in the void. Once you have mastered this you can protect your tummy from any further over-stretch and you will be less prone to further injury. Often I hear women say, 'Won't tummy exercises make it worse?' and I regularly see clients who have been avoiding any abdominal exercises, because they are worried about worsening their separation. Creating tension at your midline, your linea alba, is the answer to this. When you have built a strong and therefore stable linea alba you can return to other abdominal exercises, but not before achieving this (if you haven't done so already take a break and practise task 12 on page 157).

- Pain relief: When there is pain and inflammation our muscles cannot work so well. The inflammatory soup our body makes during the healing process means that the messages which make our muscles work cannot get through. This leads to inhibition – switching muscles off. So if you have back, pelvic, tummy, pelvic floor or rib pain this can affect your core strength and tummy recovery. I urge you to start with a visit to your GP who can discuss pain relief and/or anti-inflammatories with you. These are not to mask the problem, but to treat the root cause and get you feeling stronger quicker. Your GP can also refer you to a physiotherapist or you can see a physio, chiropractor or osteopath privately without a referral or through private medical cover. Try not to sit on it (excuse the pun!). The quicker you get the pain fixed the less likely it is your muscles will suffer.

- Avoid bloating and constipation: With all this work being put into healing, your posture and your strength, regular bulging of your belly can destabilise all that hard effort you've put in. When there is excessive gas inside the abdomen the tummy can swell and feel painful. This can also happen when movement through the digestive tract is sluggish due to food intolerances or sensitivities. Chapter 10 has all you need to know about cutting out this painful and gassy situation.

These protect steps go hand in hand with the stabilise and rehabilitation phases. Overall recovery is more than just exercise, so take from here what works for you and stick with it.

Stabilise

It is a normal strategy for our bodies to compensate for muscle weakness or injury by calling upon another muscle to do the job. When we are post-natal, with or without DRAM, the muscles at our waist can often compensate for abdominal muscle weakness at the front. If we are stiff in places, have poor posture or pain, it can make it difficult to fire up our 'core', making compensations and adaptations to our movements more likely.

If we think back to the four walls of our house and we take one away, the remaining three have to carry the load and support the building on their own. If our front tummy muscles are weakened, stretched or injured then it is normal for our waist and back to tighten up and work more.

While this sounds clever it can prove a real hindrance to regaining tension at the front, as the waist and back can dominate and take over. Therefore, you may need to start by releasing the tight pull of the obliques at your waist and spinal muscles at your back to allow the front tummy muscles to close and achieve stability. Try the first exercise below. It may surprise you how much easier it is to find and feel the tension when you have freed up what is tight and holding you back.

TASK 13 PUSH IN A WORLD OF PULL

KIT YOU WILL NEED: A massage or trigger point ball.

Low back release:

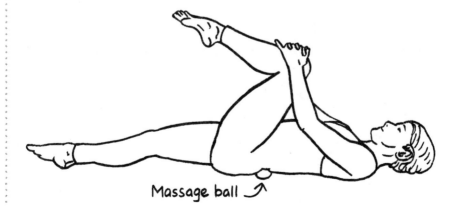

Massage ball ↗

These trigger point balls are great for getting into places! They feel like expert thumbs loosening hard-to-reach knots of muscle. Lie with one or ideally two balls underneath your lower back. One on the left, one on the right, half-way between your spine and your waist. Hug one leg in towards you and rock it forwards and back. At first it may feel tender as your back is massaged into the ball, but within 90 seconds this should ease and your back should feel more relaxed. Repeat on each side x2-3.

Mid back release:

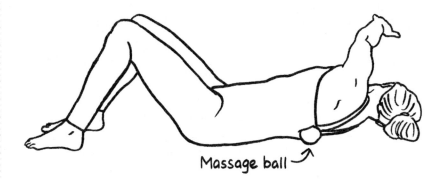

Massage ball

Often DRAM is associated with an increase in the circumference of our rib cage, which has stretched outward to accommodate our growing baby. This technique works well to mobilise those ribs, making it easier to close them again. Place a pillow under your head and find your lowest few ribs at the front and trace them around to your back. You'll feel a ridge of muscle before you get to your spine. Place the balls here and try to relax over them, using the weight of your body to apply the pressure to release these hard-working muscles. If it feels OK to do so, add in some arm hugs or overhead arms to stretch the muscle at the same time. Spend up to 90 seconds here then try moving the balls up or down to another spot that needs releasing and repeat this.

Oblique massage:

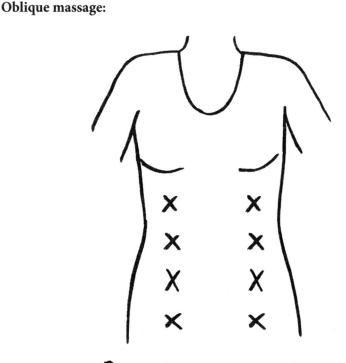

Points to press marked X

Both massage and trigger points can be done on your own tummy yourself. You want to target the outside thirds of the tummy and massage in a clockwise direction, so that you go with the direction of your gut, pressing firmly and massaging up on the right-hand wall and down on the left. At any firm and painful spots stop and press down. You may feel the discomfort radiate out or move around. These are called trigger points – 'knots' in muscles at the centre of that muscle's contraction. If you can release these you will notice an almost instant change in muscle tone. Hold your pressure down on these sore spots with one or two fingers for up to 90 seconds until they ease. If they don't ease find another nearby tender point to help release muscle tightness. You can use a massage ball instead of your hands or visit a massage therapist or physio to do this for you if you find it too sore or awkward. Work on this daily for just a few minutes alongside your exercise rehabilitation.

If you think about squeezing a balloon really hard at its waist, the pressure inside the balloon builds and pushes the contents of the balloon out at the top and bottom. Keep increasing the pressure and eventually the balloon pops. A similar thing can happen inside our tummies when our waist and back are too tense (minus the popping!). They can squeeze our waist just like the balloon and raise what is called our intra-abdominal pressure (IAP) – the pressure inside our abdomen. When our IAP builds, if there isn't enough strength at the front everything pushes up, down or out. This can give our tummy that pregnant shape even when we aren't pregnant, as well as putting pressure on our pelvic floor, increasing the risk of pelvic organ prolapse and incontinence. In this position it's hard to create tension at the midline and pelvic floor to strengthen the corset, so the waist becomes tighter to compensate and it's a vicious cycle. Break it by releasing your pesky, dominant, stronger or tighter muscles with task 13.

Most women I work with either have a *pulling* DRAM or a *passive* one. Passive ones are the easiest ones to fix as it's just a matter of strengthening, but when the tummy is being pulled apart in places by tight muscles then we have to undo the tightness before we can even consider strengthening. In a pulling DRAM the tummy continues to protrude and take on a pregnancy shape as the stronger oblique muscles pull at the waist and build pressure within the abdomen. As the front wall is weaker than the strong waist muscles, this pressure pushes everything out front. The rounded tummy is often firm to touch as it's under pressure from within. When this is the case you may be able to see the definition of your obliques at your side when you move or even when you are rested.

These may have maintained their tone and strength through your pregnancy and 'snapped back' even when the front of your tummy did not, so now the obliques are engaging in every activity, dominating movement patterns and creating further stress, stretch and instability in your front wall. They tug on the rectus muscles, pulling them out to the sides and stretch the interconnecting linea alba further. In these cases it is a miracle what oblique release can do. By manually stretching out these tightened muscles you take the strain off the front wall. Taking off the tight obliques releases the rectus muscles from their sideways pull, allowing them to slide back together.

I have treated women with 5cm and larger DRAMs and seen this drop to 1-2cm after oblique release alone, because taking the pull off allows the rectus muscles to ping back into place. This is particularly important and common when a DRAM is not new. Years after injury your body will have worked out its own compensatory ways of moving, often using the stronger waist muscles over the weakened anterior wall, and so release work is needed to reset the muscle tension more evenly. Task 13 takes you through this technique step by step.

If I had a magic wand it would probably be made of tape. It is pure magic for creating the stability we lack after any muscle injury. As I've mentioned before, it's like wearing a cast on a broken arm, because in order for the two bony ends to re-join, new bone to form between them and knit the ends together, they need to be held still. If you constantly move the two bone ends they will never heal or at best they will heal distorted. Torn or separated muscles are the same, be it in the tummy or anywhere else in the body. Every time we move – roll over in bed, get out of bed, bend down, stand back up, walk, lift the buggy, run and so on – we put strain on the healing muscle. If the linea alba does not have enough tension yet, then the two muscles can be pulled away from one another just by these everyday actions. Of course, not all of us need to tape and in most cases we are stable enough to heal without it. My two criteria for taping are:

- A gap of more than 3cm – the wider the gap the more likely the muscles will need some help coming together.
- An overstretch – when the muscles can be moved apart and the distance between them can be increased with added pressure or weight. I test this in my clinic with my client lying down and I gently stretch their muscles apart with my hands. Do they stay put or do they give? If it's the latter then it's very likely they give and stretch apart with everyday tasks too and would benefit from some support.

And it's as simple as that. It doesn't matter how post-natal you are, how old your children are, what type of delivery you had or how many pregnancies you've been through. If these two factors are present and you haven't yet tried taping, tape!

Just like that cast on your broken arm it is important to tape for long enough to allow the muscles to heal and the linea alba to thicken. I recommend six to twelve weeks as a minimum. You can, of course, continue to tape beyond this time and I often recommend applying the tape when you increase your activity or start something new. Anything explosive or high intensity – such as weightlifting, acrobatics, contact sports – puts the midline muscle under considerably more stress than everyday movements, so it's a good idea to tape for this, even when you no longer need the tape every day. I regularly recommend mums wanting to run who have DRAM or tummy weakness and pelvic floor symptoms tape just for this, to make this challenge manageable.

TASK 14 MAGIC TAPE

Search online and you'll find many taping techniques, but these two are my tried and tested favourites. The first is the most supportive and my preference as it anchors to the skeleton, just like the muscles, but if you are sensitive to tape the second alternative is just bridging the gap, anchoring from muscle to muscle, forming a second layer to the linea alba to give it some defence against overstretching.

KIT YOU WILL NEED: Stretchy kinesio tape – Rocktape is my favourite as it stays put, stretches just enough before pulling tight, rarely causes a skin reaction and comes in amazing colours (and if you're going to wear this stuff for 12 weeks that really matters!) – and a second pair of hands.

This is how you do it:

- The best place to apply the tape is lying down, as the abdominal contents move away from the stretched muscles and the tummy is at its 'flattest'. Ideally ask someone to do this for you so that you do not need to lift your head. Alternatively, use a few pillows so that you can see without needing to do a sit-up.

- Locate the bony crest of your pelvis bones and your bottom few ribs on each side.

- Cut four lengths of tape that are roughly the same length as the distance from your pelvis bone to your ribs when laid flat.

- Always apply the tape from bottom upwards so that the tape creates an up and inward action (rather than down and out).
- Start by placing the tape down across the outside rim of one pelvis bone and hold this down with one hand. Then pull the tape taught and stretch it across the tummy up towards the opposite rib cage.
- At the same time, as you lay the tape down, create as much tension at the linea alba as you can with your best cue from task 12 (see page 157), as though you're taping in the tension.
- Smooth the taut tape across your tummy, then place the ends across your ribs without tension on.
- The next piece of tape starts from the other pelvis bone.
- This is the tricky bit, because you want to cross the tape over exactly where your DRAM lies – whether this is below, above or at your navel – this is precisely where you need the tape to overlap. Place this second strip down in the same way as the first.
- Repeat this with the next two strips of tape, either above or below the first two strips, depending on where your DRAM lies. You want the four strips to cover it completely.
- Ensure these second two strips overlap the first two by several millimetres.
- I recommend using four strips of tape to start with and you can drop down to just two as your DRAM shortens in length (your gap will close like a zipper on a coat, from bottom to top pulling the sides in with it).
- When you stand up you should feel supported. Smooth out any creases in your skin under the tape as these can become sore if left creased.

Tummy taping techniques

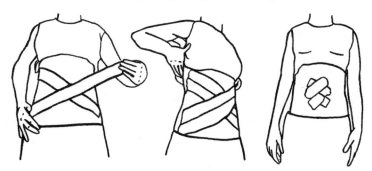

If you have sensitive skin:

- Use the same application and cross-hatching technique as above, but this time cover much less of the tummy.

- You want the tape to cover the central third of the tummy and the length of the DRAM.

- Cut six short strips of tape the width of the middle third of your tummy when it's laid horizontal.

- Start from the bottom of your DRAM moving upwards, as though you're zipping it up like a pair of jeans.

- Apply the tape from one rectus muscle diagonally up and across to the other rectus muscle.

- Alternate sides until the midline gap is covered. Depending on the length of the separation you may need less or more than six strips in total (but keep to even numbers so there is even pull on both sides).

Keep the tape on for three days and off for one day. On the off day moisturise your tummy regularly with a natural oil to ensure the skin tolerates taping well. So three days on, one day's rest, for six to 12 weeks means reapplying the tape just twice a week. You can get Rocktape wet in the shower and it doesn't affect it at all, but I would avoid soaking in the bath on taping days.

It's really important to apply these principles of protect and stabilise while you rehabilitate and not wait for them to fix the problem. Keep taping to get the most from your exercises and ensure your back and ribs stay mobile enough to achieve their full range of motion, stick to your non-bloating diet (see page 196) and maintain your good posture, all while working on these next exercises.

Rehabilitate

Any search engine will quickly provide you with hundreds of 'tummy strengthening' exercises, but not all will do what they promise! Believe it or not Dr Google doesn't have a medical qualification, nor the skills to distinguish between your tummy and anyone else's. This is not a one size fits all scenario. There are lots of factors to take into account. Many abdominal exercises, even when they're performed to the best of your ability, will use only, or mainly, the muscles at your waist, which are too far away from the problem area to make any positive difference to your midline! This is why DRAM training must be uniquely tailored. Every exercise you do to rehabilitate DRAM must create tension at your midline or else you are strengthening everything except your injury.

Pay close attention to maintain tension at your linea alba throughout your rehabilitation and keep control in all your movements. Don't be tempted to rush through the rehabilitation and attempt to do all the exercises all the time. That isn't the goal. The goal is to build on your midline tension, layer by layer, as though you are building a multi-tiered cake, encouraging healing, controlling excessive or compensatory movements, restoring strength and repeating this over and over to create tissue changes. You should see no doming (bulging out of your tummy), no 'triangle tummy' or bumps rising up and sticking out at your midline, and you shouldn't see the opposite either, so no sucking in or sinking of your midline. You need to challenge the tummy muscles to create a change and, like any recovery programme, this is measured and progressive.

TASK 15 COMPLETE DRAM RECOVERY

Don't start this series until at least six weeks post-partum or post-surgery and not until you have completed all the previous strategies in this chapter. This is not the starting point, but the rehabilitation strategy to rebuild your muscles once you are ready and stable.

The most important part is that every exercise should build your tension and narrow your gap. If this doesn't happen then you're not yet ready for that level. Only move up the levels when you are certain this is happening. Know that it takes three months to grow bigger muscles. You can progress when you're ready to progress, when you're stronger, not because of the passing of time. Keep your form, keep your patience and keep going!

KIT YOU WILL NEED: Soft Pilates ball (of course!) and a watch or timer.

These exercises are progressive, meaning they get harder, which is why they're numbered. Move on only when you feel strong enough to. Work through the ones which you feel able to do, one after the other, and stop when you struggle to achieve the position, repetitions or time. Work on all of the exercises in this sequence up to the one you're finding challenging. Work on these three to five times a week to gain strength. When you can do these well, pick up the next exercise in the sequence and drop the easiest. Keep going like this, working on a series of at least four exercises at a time, adding a harder one (a higher number on the list) and dropping the easiest on your list (the lowest number) until you've reached number 10.

Always work on at least four exercises. If you can only do the first one, or the first and second one to begin with, that's totally OK. Repeat these so that you are always doing at least four of something, even if it's exercise 1, four times. Do as many as you can but at least four each time. Aim to work continuously on each exercise for 2 minutes. You can break the 2 minutes down into manageable chunks, for example 30 seconds x4, and build your endurance as your strength builds.

The most important part of all of these is holding tension at your tummy throughout, so you must have mastered this with task 12 (see page 157), and use your technique throughout with these exercises.

1. Overhead arms in high kneeling: In a kneeling position squeeze the ball between your thighs and grow as tall as you can. Breathe out as you raise your arms above your head. Keep hold of your ribs and don't let them flare forwards as your arms move upwards. This way you'll feel your tummy tension build even more as your arms rise up. Breathe in to lower your arms and then repeat.

2. Four point press-ups:

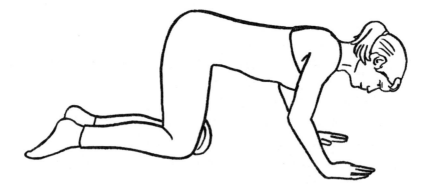

On your hands and knees, hold the ball between your thighs and create a neutral spine, maintain this throughout. Bend your elbows into a press-up as you breathe in. On your outbreath create the tummy tension and 'zip up' as you squeeze hard on the ball and press up. Repeat.

3. Half forearm plank:

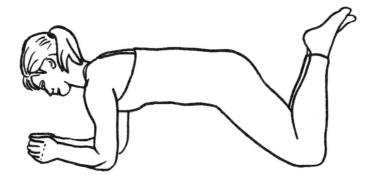

The challenge here is to hold the tension throughout. Start lying on your tummy propped up on your forearms. Maintain a neutral spine and squeeze the ball at your knees as you lift your body and hips up off the floor into a half plank and hold. There should be a straight line from your ear through your shoulder to your hip. Keep lifted through your ribs to create a gap underneath you big enough for your baby to crawl through. Don't forget to breathe.

4. Half plank press-ups:

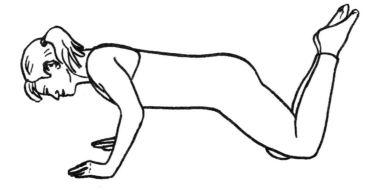

Start on your hands and knees and keep a neutral spine as you walk your hands forwards until your body and legs make one straight line with no bend in your hips. As this is more of a challenge, you want to feel that matched with more tension at your midline. Breathe in and bend your elbows lowering your body towards the mat, just as far as you can without changing your neutral spine, then breathe out, press up and squeeze the ball as you straighten your arms. Don't let your ribs stick out and really engage your tummy muscle corset. Repeat.

5. Supine lift and lower: As we move to one-sided exercises, ensure the muscles at your waist and obliques don't take the opportunity to work – instead keep the tension at your midline and your spine in neutral. From lying on your back with your knees bent, raise one leg then straighten it so that your toes are pointing to the sky. Zip up your tummy and exhale as you lower your leg to the floor. Inhale and raise the leg. Spend 1 minute on each leg. Try not to let the rest of your body move or change shape, just your leg.

6. Table top squeeze: My favourite exercise! From lying with your knees bent, raise one leg off the ground, bending your hip and knee to right angles. As you create tension and zip up your tummy, raise your second leg to join your first. Place the ball between your knees and squeeze it as you breathe, keeping tension through your tummy and your spine in neutral. Use the weight of your legs and squeeze of the ball to close your tummy from the sides in. Keep tension on throughout to stop your tummy doming outwards. Hold and breathe.

7. Table top hip twist: Another challenge to target the weakness at your midline without your obliques overworking. Lie down and raise your legs to table top, one at a time as per exercise 6. Keep one of your legs completely still as the other rolls out to the side from the hip. Encourage your outbreath and tummy tension to build even more as your leg moves in. Alternate legs and be sure to only roll from your hip – your bottom should stay level with your pelvis grounded to the floor. As one leg rolls out be sure not to allow the other side of your pelvis to lift up.

8. Curl ups: This is the first exercise to shorten the rectus abdominis at the front of your tummy – a challenge but one you've built up to. You're not going up or down as this would move the muscle too much. Lie on your back with both knees bent, the ball between your knees and your feet on the floor. Next, raise your head and shoulders up from the floor and hold it there, sliding your ribs down towards your pelvis and keeping your lower back and pelvis in neutral. It's important to watch your tummy draw in when you set your tension and keep it here as you curl up to the ceiling, not down to your knees. Hold and squeeze the ball.

9. Table top curl up: From lying, raise your legs to table top one at a time and then squeeze the ball between your knees. Focus on lifting your arms and shoulders up to the ceiling, not crunching down towards your knees as your head and shoulders lift up away from the floor and curl up. Keep your tummy in by holding tension and continuing to squeeze the ball at your knees. Breathe and hold this as long as you can. Rest when you need to, but spend 2 minutes on this. Aim to hold for 15 seconds x8.

10. Box planks: Start on your hands and knees. Find a flat back position to shorten your tummy muscles and then tuck your toes under. As you breathe keep midline tension as you press into the floor and hover your knees just a few inches away from the ground. Maintain a flat back with your tail out and squeeze the ball at your knees. Don't forget to breathe and hold as long as you can. Rest when you need to, but spend 2 minutes on this. Aim to hold for 15 second x8.

You may find that you work through this task but still need more strength in order to achieve your goals. To keep building strength you need to keep building the pressure or what physios call 'the load'. These next exercises do just that. Again, the most important part is to maintain tension throughout. Work on these in a series, one after the other, to get the muscle changes you need. Just to stress, these are advanced tummy exercises, NOT a starting point. Add these in at the very end, once you have completed numbers 1 to 10 with great form and need some extra levels. Don't rush ahead and feel you need to get to these – it's much more helpful to do the previous exercises well.

For extra abdominal strength, aim to work hard for 30 seconds, rest for 10 seconds maximum and then repeat four times for each exercise. Your target is to work on at least four exercises in every session and include exercises from 1 to 10 if you need to. This means your programme may be anything from 7 to 11 to 11 to 15, depending on how far you've progressed.

11. Full plank:

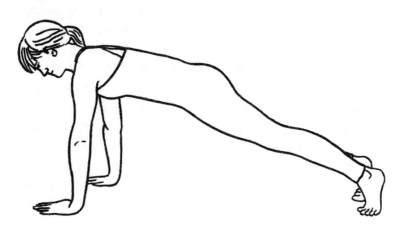

Start on your hands and knees with your hands out at the top of your mat. Find a neutral spine and first create tension, on your outbreath lift and hover your knees, then send your legs straight to find a full plank position. Hold your form here. If you can't quite make 30 seconds break this down and perhaps try holding 15 seconds x8.

12. Toe taps in curl up: Start in lying and your legs to table top one at a time, keeping tension in your tummy as you do. Then feel the tension build as you curl your head and shoulders up off the floor, holding your lower back in neutral. Breathe out and lower one leg to tap your toes on your mat, breathe in as it comes back up and you return to table top. Then repeat on the opposite leg. Maintain your curl up and tummy tension for as many repetitions as you can, alternating sides.

13. Single leg stretch in curl up: And the load keeps going up! Don't compromise your midline, instead make the tension build and your tummy draw in throughout this exercise. Start in table-top and raise your head and shoulders up off the floor to curl up maintaining tension through your tummy and no doming. Then reach one leg out straight on your outbreath and feel your tension build. Hold this as the leg comes back in and then change sides. Alternate your leg stretches on each outbreath, holding your curl up. Reset as many times as you need to keep your form throughout the 2 minutes.

14. Plank with arm raises: Find your full plank position as in exercise 11. From here, squeeze a ball between your knees, maintain a neutral spine and tummy tension as you reach one arm forwards on your outbreath. Lower your arm back down to the mat as you breathe in but maintain your form and tension, no resting! Alternate your arm raises for as long as you can, trying to hold for longer each time before your need to rest and reset for a real challenge.

15. Curl up, double leg stretch: Start in table top before you lift your head and shoulders to the sky, maintaining your tummy tension. Breathe out as you squeeze a ball between your knees and reach your legs away from you, straightening your knees. Breathe in as they fold back to table top, then repeat. Don't let your back lift up away from the mat, instead hold your neutral spine. This will dictate how low your legs go. If your back starts to lift then your legs are going too low and instead when you straighten them away from you take them higher. Keep the tension and don't let your tummy change shape throughout this challenge.

When you get to this point you will have built sufficient tension for most tasks, but all these exercises are very controlled and static, and that's why we start here. The next part is to incorporate normal movement. We need our tummy muscles to work as we move in and out of positions, to wind up and shorten, then release and lengthen with control. Often I see women who have been doing bicycle crunches (where you curl up and twist from side to side while moving alternate legs out straight) or heel taps (holding a curl up and touching alternating heels with their finger tips, side bending their waist) in a misguided attempt to recover their DRAM. These exercises all move us too much for healing to happen, but instead are challenges for much later. They can be introduced at the final hurdle and only if we need to. Ease back into the exercise, sport and challenges you enjoy as you continue to strengthen.

If you struggle to progress your strength and move up through the different levels of this task, you may need to take one step back to keep moving forward. Look back at task 11 on page 143, tick these exercises off and then come back to tummy rebuilding. It may be that your skeleton, your scaffolding, needs putting in place first before you can fix your muscles with any success.

However, it's important to know that whenever you start to try to heal your DRAM or natural tummy muscle stretch it is never too late. I often meet mothers of grown-up children who assume they've missed the boat and that it's too late to address their tummy strength and changes that date back to their pregnancies. To them I say, 'How do you know? Is it not worth a try?' One study asked physios about their experiences in supporting women who had been living with DRAM for more than two years and specifically if there was still the opportunity for improvement. Every physio agreed that there is some degree of recovery, whether you start retraining at six, 60 or 600+ weeks post-pregnancy and birth.

When is it past the point of no return?

If I struggle to feel any tension at the midline when I'm examining for DRAM, despite trying all my tricks and ball squeezing exercises, then I scan the client with our ultrasound machine. While an expert's assessment using just the hands is as clear as what we see in diagnostic ultrasound, I often use this to double-check and confirm, or not, what I am feeling. On ultrasound I am looking for the distinctive white line of the linea alba bridging the midline. Sometimes it is only visible in parts and not along the whole length of the midline. I recommend these women to pursue rehab regardless. If we work on the portion of the midline that is intact and where we do have tension, then we can bring the void together. We may not close it completely, but it will be much less noticeable when reduced. Remember the coat zipper? It may not be fully zipped, but it is a lot more closed and together than it was before.

If the gap is more than five fingers apart, there is no tension and I can see no linea alba on the ultrasound it is likely we will be able to see and feel the internal organs pressing through. In this instance, the rehab potential is limited. However, when I'm working with women at this stage I always try my whole catalogue of exercises to see if a glimmer of tension can be summoned. In my whole career only a few women didn't have this and they went on to have surgical repairs. This is where the muscles on either side are stitched together, sometimes using a mesh to bridge the gap. This surgery is pretty successful, but the recovery period is long and slow. Like any abdominal surgery there is no lifting for six to 12 weeks, including your babies. Most surgeons would encourage you to wait for at least two years post-birth before considering this option as your body needs this time to recover from pregnancy as a whole. But this time can be used to build strength and stability in all other areas affected by pregnancy and birth, so that a tummy repair has the best chance of success. If the front wall is repaired without healing and rebuilding the foundations, floor, walls and roof, then the surgery may not be as successful as it could be.

Real-life story

Susie, mum of three girls, went from split down the middle to stronger than ever

Being pregnant with and giving birth to twins was the hardest thing I have ever done. What hadn't really occurred to me was that after they were born my body might not spring back quite as quickly as it had after my first child. The twins were born at 36 weeks weighing in at an impressive 6lbs 5oz and 6lbs 2oz – a combined weight of 12lbs 7oz – so it's no wonder I could barely walk in the run-up to their birth! When my labour started spontaneously I went to hospital for a planned Caesarean section, which was deemed the safest delivery for me and my twins. I recovered well but by seven weeks, when everything else had healed, it became clear that my tummy muscles had not. The rest of my body was looking relatively normal, but my stomach felt very weak and sagged in the middle.

A physio assessment and ultrasound scan (also done by my physio at the same time) revealed a severe DRAM of more than 5cm running all the way up from my Caesarean scar to my ribs. It was good to get a proper diagnosis, but I also felt devasted. After a very tough twin pregnancy I wanted to feel and look 'normal' again, and, most importantly, to get back to the exercise that I loved.

Eager to fix this I took in all my options, including paying privately for surgery to knit the two sides of my stomach back together. As it stood, I was effectively at risk of my insides falling out through the middle. Yuck! The surgeon was of the opinion that no amount of rehab was going to solve my problem and surgery was my only option… which felt like another blow. But I was determined to throw myself into doing what I could naturally and decided to give myself two years to get as strong as I could be through physiotherapy and exercise. Besides, surgery, or more importantly the six to 12-week recovery period where I couldn't lift my babies, was not an option for me as a new mum of three.

With the support of tape to effectively hold me together as I healed, I stuck to my rebuilding plan and did about 25 minutes of gentle exercises every day. This was really hard to find time for with newborn twins and a three-year-old, but I was encouraged by seeing results that my physio confirmed in just three weeks! So that was the start. I would work hard at home and every three weeks my physio would give me a new set of exercises which progressively got more advanced. Progress did feel painfully slow, but very gradually I started to feel stronger and visually things were improving. After nine weeks I'd managed to reduce the gap to about 2-3cm – just at my belly button – and it had closed to just a few millimetres above and below. I no longer had a 12cm split!

I'm now 13 months post-partum and I feel strong and proud of how far I've come. I can do most advanced Pilates and there are only a few exercises which I feel are very tough still. I'm not having to do the rehab every day anymore – more like three times a week – and I'm confident that I won't need any surgery. I'm hoping that over the next year I might recover even more and even forget the gap was ever there!

When to ask for help:

- If you can see lumps and bump rising up from your midline and you suspect you have a hernia. While not all of these require medical attention, if they are painful of causing you concern it is a very valid reason to visit your doctor.

- When you are unable to progress through these tasks, see your tummy doming outwards or caving in even while using this guide, or just need some extra guidance or support for finding and achieving tension.

- You have back pain, leaking or pelvic organ prolapse that you suspect is related to DRAM and it has not resolved despite the exercises in this book.

What to ask for:

- Women's health physiotherapy in the first instance. You can start treatment and the healing and rebuilding journey can begin straightaway. Even if other investigations are also needed these can be done alongside your physical therapy. Note: it's very important to ensure the physio you are referred to has experience with DRAM. Some women's health physios are experts in incontinence, others in pelvic girdle pain. Not all are experts on your tummy, so it's vital to establish that you have been referred to the right expert for your problem.

- An ultrasound scan if you suspect or know that you have a hernia. This is performed by a sonographer at a hospital and is the same machine used to take a look at your baby through your pregnancy. A grainy black and white image will reveal to the sonographer if there is a true hernia (the bowel is pushing through), the size (and therefore potential for avoiding surgery) and if there is any immediate risk to your organs (anything getting trapped that would need urgent attention). Even if there is no need for surgical treatment it is still important to discuss the findings with your doctor to find a non-surgical solution and be directed to a physiotherapist for protect, stabilise and rehabilitate strategies.

- A referral to a general surgeon or advice on private surgical options. Hernia repair is currently offered in the UK with the NHS, but DRAM repair (a procedure called abdominoplasty) is not, unless you have significant other injuries as a result. I've worked with several women whose back pain and leaking symptoms didn't resolve despite physiotherapy because their DRAM was too severe. Without this support at the front of their cylinder they were unable to restore strength in the rest. These women went on to have surgical DRAM repair with the NHS and all had successful resolution of their back pain and leakiness as a result. There is also a private route you can take if you want to have your tummy split repaired, but in either instance you must complete a course of physiotherapy first to ensure you have the strength, skills and understanding to heal and rebuild after surgery.

What's important

- After pregnancy all women will have a relative stretch weakness of their tummy muscles. This needs rehabilitating.
- In addition to regular stretch weakness, one third of us will also have true abdominal muscle separation – DRAM. This definitely needs rehabilitating.

- Rehabilitation does not just include exercise, but positioning and postural changes too. It may be the missing piece in your puzzle.
- Even chronic DRAM can benefit from healing and rebuilding. It's never too late.
- Release any muscles and tightness which is not serving you. Equip yourself with the tools to do this yourself.
- It's not all about the width of the gap. Creating tension across depth is the measure of success with tummy muscle recovery and step one in recovering a DRAM.
- Don't be tempted to skip straight to the hardest tummy strengthening exercises. Slow and steady, incorporating all the elements of protect, stabilise and rehabilitate is the best way to heal and rebuild safely.
- DRAM recovery must include abdominal muscle loading. Once you can create tension at your midline you can stabilise the DRAM and work on closing the distance with strength-based exercise.

9. Breathing: Firing up your engine

When you consider that we take around 20,000 breaths a day and have done since the day we were born it sounds like the most natural thing in the world, yet so many of us are left wondering if our bodies have forgotten how to breathe normally after pregnancy and birth. It would be a huge effort to be aware of every breath we took – imagine it: 20,000 conscious manoeuvres before we've done anything else, even while we sleep! – but re-learning how to breathe with the least effort and the right body parts goes hand in hand with the recovery of everything we have discussed so far. It sounds complicated and it's easy to get tangled up in knots when you're trying to master breathing properly. How should we breathe exactly? Should we use our tummy muscles? What about our pelvic floor? Should we practise lying down or standing up? Does yoga count? So let's start at the beginning and look at changes that happen to our bodies in pregnancy. If we understand the picture and what the puzzle should look like it is much easier to rebuild.

First trimester

- In weeks 2 to 5 we see our heart rate increase by 16 to 20 beats per minute, often before we even know we are expecting. As our body demands more oxygen and our heart works harder, our breathing rate also increases. It's very common to feel short of breath at the slightest exertion and to be gasping for air even in those early weeks. This is an outward sign of all the amazing changes happening under our skin.

- The hormones relaxin and progesterone increase to prepare our womb for embryo implantation by relaxing its muscles, preventing early contractions, as well as supporting growth of the placenta. However, the problem is that like all hormones they cannot act on just one part of us and our whole body experiences their effects. This means our blood vessels dilate, dropping our blood pressure; our gut relaxes and digestion feels slower, and our muscles and joints stretch more. This trilogy of normal pregnancy adaptations

185

can give rise to injury and early discomfort, especially with breathing. We may notice rib or mid-back pain as the joints here move more with each breath we take, or we may find it takes an increased effort to breathe in and contract our diaphragm from its new lengthened, relaxed position.

Second trimester

- As our body and growing baby continue to demand more oxygen we take in 30-40% more air with every breath we take. You might notice that you're panting even with the slightest exertion as you are already breathing 30-40% harder just at rest!

- Relaxin reaches its peak in trimester 2, which is when pelvic, back and rib pain are more likely, especially as your baby bump emerges and adds further to the weight to be carried by these areas.

- Progesterone's relaxing effect on the smooth muscle of our digestive tract, combined with the 'squish' which starts in this trimester as our baby seems to take over our abdomen, can result in painful reflux. This is where the acidic contents of our stomach move back up the oesophagus as the muscle valves between the two organs do not close fully. We may also experience constipation as everything tends to stick around for a lot longer, which is our body's way of ensuring every last nutrient is absorbed for you and your baby. Our digestion can feel sluggish at best. The discomfort of this can change our movement and also our breath patterns, with often more shallow breathing, sometimes breath holding, and straining to push out a poo.

Third trimester

- As our baby seems to fill our entire abdomen our ability to take a full breath in is down by 20% as we have less space to breathe deeply.

- As our baby reaches full term our diaphragm is pushed upwards and our ribcage is forced outwards by 4cm or more. This is annoying on more levels than just needing to buy new bras. While it doesn't sound like a lot, imagine moving your front door 4cm up from its hinges or stretching its door frame out by 4cm. Things are going to get pretty draughty and good luck shutting the door! When you consider the building analogy, it's no wonder incontinence while pregnant is a common complaint and, like the door to our houses and the walls beyond, each part of our abdominal cylinder is interconnected.

- 10-15kg of total weight gain is expected and easy to reach when you add up:
  - Baby 3.5kg (or thereabouts)
  - Placenta 1kg (seriously, did you see that thing?!)
  - Breast growth of up to 1kg (while it feels like more, it's normally only half a kilo each, but just think about that next time you pick up a bag of flour – that's a lot of weight to stuff down our bra!)
  - Fluid 3.6kg (this is made up from extra blood volume, amniotic fluid around our baby and also just fluid floating around our cells making us puffy)
  - ...and already we're at 9.1kg without even starting to eat for two!

Just this on its own goes a long way to understanding why breathing feels so different now. Suddenly we are drawing in air for 10-15kg more of us.

Despite knowing these anatomical and mechanical changes, the effort it took to take a full breath in, speak or to climb stairs was a shock to me in both my pregnancies. The conscious gasping for air initially amused both me and my husband, until it became painful and frustrating, which I'm sure you can relate to.

Pregnancy posture and breathing

With all these pregnancy changes there are inevitable changes to our posture, so let's recap the two most common postures in pregnancy and post-birth: sway and lordotic.

In sway posture we round our shoulders forwards and our ribcage and diaphragm sink down. This shrinks the space inside our lungs for precious air to fill. Instead of filling up most of our lung space with our normal 12 breaths a minute, we need to breathe much more frequently to get the same amount of oxygen into our body's many muscles. Our diaphragm struggles to pull our breath in from this cramped position and we need to use the smaller muscles in our neck instead. These neck muscles were not built to take on this task single-handedly and soon become tired and painful, making breathing more of an effort still.

In lordotic posture our rib cage flares forwards, stretching our diaphragm and tummy muscles. While this gives us more space to breathe than in sway posture, these muscles need to work harder from here to contract, shorten and pull air in. The extra effort required raises the pressure inside our abdomen so that it is tense most of the time. Like the walls of a balloon which is filled to capacity, the pressure from the air inside stretches the walls almost to bursting point. This is not a problem if we have a back and pelvic floor strong enough to tolerate this, but it can lead to incontinence, prolapse, back pain and DRAM if there is an injury, or weakness in any part of the abdominal cylinder.

So optimal posture can help with optimal breathing, and when we find our best posture, breathing correctly follows easily. Go back and do task 2 (see page 39) if you think yours could still do with some TLC.

The muscles at the floor (pelvic floor) and the roof (diaphragm) of our abdomen work in sync and, just as in other things we take for granted (like going for a poo), we rarely consider how breathing works until it doesn't. The pelvic floor, diaphragm and muscular walls of the abdominal cylinder both impact on and are impacted by the strength of one another. You may not be conscious of this normally, but when there is pain, injury or weakness you can become acutely aware of the difficulties breathing poses to your pelvic strength. With each breath in and as the lungs fill, the pressure inside our tummy builds, creating down and outward forces on the abdominal muscles and the pelvic floor. If they are not strong enough to resist and push back, we may experience leaking, tummy bulging or feeling that 'everything is falling out'.

Similarly, when you breathe out the diaphragm retracts and lifts upwards. So does your pelvic floor and the pressure inside of us goes down. This moment of breathing out is the best time to work on your strength, when you have the least resistance or pressure to work against. You can use this upward movement of your diaphragm when you breathe out to help you raise the pelvic organs and your pelvic floor, just as you practised in task 4 (see page 58).

However, think about when we exhale – not just when we breathe out, but also when we laugh, shout, cough, blow or sing. Extra effort is needed by our tummy muscles and diaphragm to forcefully push the air out in these activities. This increases the pressure inside our abdomen once more. If the pelvic floor strength cannot match this, we will be unable to lift our bladder, kink our pee pipes and stop our pelvic organs from dropping down. We won't feel an upward lift of the pelvic floor when we need to resist the downward force, but the opposite, and again we can become painfully aware of the un-harmonious relationship between coughing or sneezing and wet knickers.

The good news is that we can train our abdominal cylinder and pelvic ring to overcome the natural changes to our breath pattern that occurred as a result of pregnancy and birth. We can then cough, laugh, sneeze and even lift heavy weights to our heart's content, confident in the knowledge that we've trained our pelvic floor to cope with these challenges.

Optimal breath

Let's remind ourselves how to breathe and restore strength and tone in our diaphragm, the roof of the pelvic floor and consequently our *house* as a whole. Our goal is that over time activities which require forceful breath, such as sneezing, singing or even just blowing our nose, will no longer leave us feeling embarrassed, self-conscious or in need of a change of clothes. Consider preparing for these events like training for a sporting event. You train the muscles to be fit for the task and you can train your abdominal cylinder in the same way, so that you can sing, laugh and sneeze as you did before, in the moment, instead of being distracted by pain and discomfort.

TASK 16 BREATHING FOR THE FIRST TIME

KIT YOU WILL NEED: Just somewhere you can focus and be still.

Before you begin, try to get into your best posture. This will allow you to access all of your muscles. Grow tall, as though your head is a balloon full of helium, floating up to the ceiling. As you've done before, imagine that you are wearing your favourite necklace and you are showing it off to the room, lifting your breastbone and allowing the necklace to shine. At the same time melt your shoulder blades down your back as though they are dripping chocolate… Try to keep this posture even when your focus drifts.

STEP 1

Use both hands to feel for your ribcage at the sides of your body, underneath your bra strap. Trace your ribs around to the front until your fingers meet and rest your palms flat against your chest wall. Take a few normal breaths and just notice what you feel. Don't try to change anything, just become aware of the movements happening beneath your hands.

Then use your next inbreath to move your fingertips apart, expanding your ribcage sideways into the palms of your hands (this may take a bit of practice). Try giving your ribcage a squeeze so that instead of resting your palms on your chest wall you're pressing them against it and pushing the air out. On your next inbreath meet this resistance. Push back against the squeeze and feel your rib cage open as you draw air in. You are using your diaphragm, and each muscle between every rib, to expand your chest wall and pull air in and down to the base of your lungs. At the same time your tummy, back and pelvic floor become taut as they tighten with the increased pressure inside your abdomen. Imagine wearing a tight corset, but instead of preventing you from breathing in it just gives you enough resistance to tighten as you expand your chest and middle.

Now let's try and slow things down. Take in the same volume of air, but lengthen the breath, giving each and every muscle the time and chance to engage, and inhale into every corner of your lungs. Try breathing in for six, slow and steady, then out for six. Keep the intensity of your inbreath and outbreath the same. This is called diaphragmatic breathing. You are breathing with your entire abdominal cylinder. Well done!

Next, try keeping this same technique, but taking more 'normal-sized' breaths for you. Try to just take in as much air as you need, but keep the movement the same, expanding your ribcage and breathing into your corset.

STEP 2

When you breathe in you should notice that your tummy gently expands when your rib cage does. Your diaphragm is moving downwards, pushing your organs down into your belly to make room for air inside your lungs. Notice how your belly doesn't feel soft, but firmer as the muscles contract and lengthen. Your pelvic floor is doing the same. You want to strengthen the muscles and practise this breath pattern so that the pelvic floor allows both the downward movement and the increased pressure while still maintaining strength and support.

Now notice that as you breathe out your tummy pulls in to push the diaphragm up and the air out of your lungs. Can you feel your pelvic floor doing the same? No? Let's practise.

Place one hand on your rib cage and one on your tummy. First get into a rhythm of diaphragmatic breathing (step 1). Your tummy will be moving a little, but your rib cage (and diaphragm) will be moving a lot. On your next inhale imagine the diaphragm pulling down and the pelvic floor doing the same. Don't push it down, just allow the breath to happen. As you breathe out, contract your pelvic floor to draw the sitting bones together. Imagine there is a string tied to each sitting bone, running towards the middle of the pelvic floor and up through the centre of your body, through the diaphragm and out of the crown of your head. As you breathe out, imagine that string being pulled gently upwards, gathering the pelvic floor, tightening the muscular diaphragms and moving them upwards. As you breathe in, let go of that string and allow the diaphragm to move downwards, so that you are slowly and with control lowering the pelvic floor back to its rest position. You should feel a gradual lengthening and release until it is relaxed. Take a few normal breaths before repeating the exercise.

Keep practicing until it feels possible for you to synchronise your outbreath with your pelvic floor contraction and your inbreath with its relaxation. This is the way our bodies naturally function, but pregnancy, childbirth, pain and injury can alter this synchronisation and it is very likely you will need to retrain it. Sequencing your breath to your pelvic floor contraction and relaxation will really help in rebuilding your body's strength, so it is worth a bit of practice here. This is a process of repetition. Practise every day and in two to four weeks your brain, nerves and muscles will learn to do this naturally. This is called motor patterning or muscle memory. I can't stress how helpful it is to take some time out to master this. Try it lying down, on all fours, standing and sitting.

Be aware, this can be a challenge to master on its own before combining it with other exercises. Women often tell me they have to hold their breath to hold their pelvic floor exercises (from task 4 on page 58) or worry when to breathe while also mastering tension at their separated tummy muscles (see task 12 on page 157). Don't worry – breathing correctly can be too difficult to combine with any other task at the beginning. Or rather, these other tasks demand all your attention to perfect so don't get tied up with also breathing correctly. Try not to worry about combining them initially, but practise each exercise on its own and combine the breathing only when you've mastered them. You'll find my instructions on when to breathe in and out and hold with every exercise, but know that combining both the action and the breath together requires patience. I am not expecting you to get it straightaway. Take time to re-learn to breathe again.

You may well have already heard of or even practised other breathing strategies to relieve pelvic floor dysfunctions, such as something called hypopressives. Hypopressive exercises are thought to reduce the pressure inside our abdomen, restore both voluntary and involuntary control of the pelvic floor, and syncronise how it works with the rest of our core muscles. In simple terms hypopressives require you to breathe out fully and hold for as long as you can before breathing in again. The truth is incorporating breath training alongside pelvic floor muscle re-training is what leads to the greatest success in reducing symptoms of incontinence and prolapse, not any one breathing exercise alone. While ensuring the body's optimal breathing pattern is restored, we also need to ensure that we have re-built strength in our tummies, backs and pelvic floors enough for life's many and varied challenges. I am a physiotherapist and my job is to enable people to move and return to what they enjoy. While breath work is an important feature, rebuilding physical strength has to be a part of this as well. There is new research coming out all the time and I will continue to keep my eye on this one, but for now remember that pelvic floor muscle retraining and breath work is most beneficial when practised *together.*

Both my brother and my father are mechanical engineers and I'd say physios are engineers too. We work out how things move and coordinate to get the most efficient, pain-free movement. What goes on below the car bonnet happens without us thinking about it until things go wrong and it's the same with breathing. Air is our first fuel, our body's life source, but breathing is something we rarely think about until it becomes more difficult. When you consider all the anatomical changes our bodies go through in each stage of pregnancy, it really is no wonder we need to re-learn and re-train our every breath.

What's important

- The pelvic floor is our building's foundations and the diaphragm is the roof. These muscles move as one, rising and falling in synch. Their strength needs to match.

- Forceful breathing, including coughing, sneezing and laughing, can lead to incontinence and pelvic organ prolapse when there is weakness or injury within the abdominal cylinder.
- Optimal posture gives way to optimal breathing. When you find your best posture, breathing follows easily.
- Train your breath to suit your challenges. Combine your breath work with what you need your body to be able to do – sing, shout, jump, lift. You get the picture.
- Combine breathing with other challenges only when you're able to. Consider each task in this book, including breathing, as a challenge in its own right. You'll be a master of your rebuilding when you can complete any task and breathing in synchronisation.

10. Fuelling your journey: What goes in must come out

A huge part of our recovery after pregnancy and birth comes down to properly fuelling ourselves to make healing, repair and rebuilding possible. We all know that any disruption to our lifestyle and daily routine can also mean changes to the way we nourish our bodies. Holidays, working from home or flexible shift patterns inevitably involve us eating at different times or consuming different amounts or different types of foods compared to our normal diet. There is no bigger change to our regular routine than having a baby! Night and day merge into one with meal times becoming more like frequent snacks and food choices prioritised by convenience. We are pulled away from our normal nutrition due to limited sleep and many of us have the added challenge of breast feeding, so our body is our baby's main source of fuel. This can play havoc with our digestion. Without our regular dietary input we can start to struggle with constipation or, the opposite, develop an irritable bowel with an increased need to go urgently, energy highs and lows, bloating and sensitive bladder issues. This can lead to pain, peeing more frequently, wanting to go to the loo all the time and sometimes not making it. Keeping a balanced diet and regular fluid intake requires planning, two free hands and having ready access to what is seasonal and nutritious. This is never more important than when healing and recovering from pregnancy and birth, and it's time to address the basics of this – our fuel.

Drink up

Our number one fuel source is water. Our bodies are 60% water and so we need to ensure that we have plenty of fluid coming in for new tissue growth and healing. Getting enough water when you have two free hands, a normal routine and no baby was a struggle, so I bet it's even more so now! If you are breast feeding you also need to drink enough water to make milk for your baby too. You should aim for 1.5 litres a day – roughly six to eight glasses. I recommend taking this like medicine, so here's your prescription:

Take 500ml three times a day, ideally with rest, to heal and feel stronger.

If you are breast feeding, also consider this: a newborn baby drinks 45-90mls every two to three hours, adding up to one litre a day. As they grow, they will need even more than this. You therefore need to account for an extra litre of fluid going in, so there is enough for the both of you.

We should also discuss the other drinks you were thinking of too. Alcohol can be a bladder irritant and can cause you to need to pee more frequently or more urgently. I'm sure you don't need me to tell you this – we've all seen and stood in the long queues for the ladies at bars and events. I'm just going to put it out there, but if your bladder isn't very happy when you've drunk alcohol you may well make a huge step in your recovery if you give it a rest for a while. And while fizzy soft drinks are tempting for a refreshing quick hit of energy too, you won't be surprised to hear they're not great for us either. The gas can leave us with painful, bloated bellies and difficulty opening our bowels. High in sugar and low in, well, anything good for us, they can leave you thirstier than before and are a poor substitute for a nice, cool glass of water.

Caffeine is another vice that may be worth cutting back on, because it can irritate and stimulate both your bladder and your bowel, and make you lurch for the bathroom. That may not be a problem unless you have post-birth injuries to consider or an ordinarily sluggish digestive system that has backed up thanks to pregnancy or those post-labour iron supplements. Caffeine is also a diuretic, which means it makes you wee more. Again, not too much of a problem if you're drinking enough water, unless you also have a new inability to hold your wee in. This is not to say that if you wet yourself you shouldn't drink coffee, but it may be a part of the problem. Think of it as the protect part of healing a weak bladder. Take away the irritant to give your bladder (and bowel) a rest while you stabilise and rehabilitate. You can always add these things back in once you have rebuilt your strength.

Avoiding the dreaded bloat

Bloating is very common and can be a result of unhappy hormones, food sensitivities or just a big delicious meal. Sometimes it is the time of day, the amount of food or certain types of food which affect us, leaving us with swollen painful tummies filled with excess gas. Big meals, eating late at night, gluten, dairy and high sugar foods are all common triggers. As well as being very uncomfortable, bloating can change our posture, the way we move, affect our bowel movements and stretch our healing tummy muscles. But prevention is always better than cure and figuring out what is causing so much upset to your insides is a better solution than just reaching for the indigestion tablets. Below are my top tips for avoiding the dreaded bloat.

- Keep a food diary to identify any triggers, that is foods that set off your stomach pain and swelling. Make a note of all that goes in and out, and the timings, as well as noting when you feel bloated. Score this from zero to ten, with zero being no discomfort and ten being the worst. You may soon start to see a pattern. For example, if dairy is your trigger, you may record a one after your cup of milky coffee, a four after your cheesy pizza and a ten after your yoghurt bowl. At first glance it may be tricky to see what the theme is, but before long you will build a picture of food groups that your tummy doesn't fancy.

- Take a pro-biotic to help your healthy bacteria reduce gas and move things through your system happily. You can find these as expensive supplements to take daily or at the supermarket in natural and kefir yoghurt. You can also make kefir at home – it's super simple with milk and some good bacteria (but please Google where to obtain 'live cultures for kefir' as any old bacteria will not do!).

- Avoid sugary fizzy drinks (including those with alcohol – sorry), beans, wheat, cabbage, onions and other gas-producing foods.

- Take a full 12-hour break from food overnight to let your tummy rest.

- Eat slowly to avoid taking in air. Again, this is not easy with a newborn when you need to stuff food in whenever you can, but if you are suffering with bloating this may be something you'll need to address.

- Ingest a few drops of peppermint oil or sip a peppermint tea to ease the pain and deflate your tum.

- Take a walk or some exercise. Movement on the outside creates movement on the inside. You might want to do this on your own or with close family as all that gas will likely move down and out along your walk!

Pump up the protein

Most quick and easy snacks (which, let's face it, is the new normal!) are high in sugars. This provides us with an instant, often much needed, kick and energy source, but one that is relatively short lived. Protein provides us with a much longer lasting supply of energy, meaning we don't feel hungry again as quickly or notice a post sugar-high dip in energy, as well as providing our body's tissues with what it needs to repair. The recommended daily allowance is 0.8g of protein per kilo per day, which is, on average, 45-55g – a whole chicken breast or two big scoops of full fat yogurt topped with seeds and nuts. This may not sound like a lot. However, when you're a new mum, often with only one free hand, finding enough protein that's easy to prepare can be a tough challenge in itself. I've met many mothers whose only daily protein sources were a scoop of humous, a milky coffee or a handful of nuts, so you may need to be resourceful here and think outside the biscuit box.

It's worth taking a look at your daily diet and ensuring there is some protein in each meal rather than all in one chunk at dinner time – shortly before you go to bed, when it is hardest to process. I appreciate weighing and measuring your food is both dull and inconvenient, and I'm not suggesting you do this religiously, but I do strongly suggest getting a rough idea of what your protein source is. Here's a quick guide that you can add your own favourites to:

Food	Protein (grams)
85g tuna, salmon, haddock or trout	21
One cooked chicken or turkey breast	19
170g plain Greek yoghurt	17
½ cup cottage cheese	14
½ cup cooked beans	8
1 cup milk (including in a milky coffee!)	8
¼ cup of nuts (all types)	7
1 egg	6

So how about scrambled eggs for breakfast, a tuna sandwich for lunch, a chicken breast salad or stew for dinner, and a delicious yoghurt pud to tick off your daily protein needs? Other great options are nut, seed or protein-based snack bars. These are becoming more readily available at convenience stores and even local garages. Look out for ones made with natural ingredients and sweetened with natural sugars so that you're only getting good fats and carbs in alongside your protein fix. These companies are missing a trick not marketing their snacks to new mums who need them the most. I vote we push these as maternity leave snacks, and leave the coffee and cake for parties!

Protein shakes are also brilliant both in pregnancy and after birth. Again, not often marketed to mothers, but more to body-builder types who, ironically, are probably already getting enough protein, gym time and all the rebuilding fuel they need! These shakes are not just for body builders, men or those wanting to 'bulk up'. Plant-based powders (such as soy and pea) are packed full of not just protein but all the essential fats, vitamins and minerals we need in the perfect, convenient package. You can prepare these and keep them in the fridge for a quick go-to one-handed snack. They were my saviour when I was pregnant with number two and morning sickness hit mid-afternoon, just in time for when I was due to collect my toddler. This slow release fuel source got me through the danger zone of nausea to dinner time (check out task 17 on page 203 for my favourite recipe).

Get fit fats

Our bodies need various types of fats for basic functions such as movement, blood clotting and reducing inflammation. Fats are the building blocks of all our hormones and without them we are prone to hormonal imbalances. They are essential for sleep, digestion and of course reproduction. Fats also boost our metabolism and promote weight loss. Yes really! But there are some fats that are not so good for us; those that drive up our cholesterol and increase our risk of heart disease. These are trans fats.

For far too long 'fat' has been associated with 'diet', but when we cut out fat we cut out some of the essential nutrients our body desperately needs. I'm sure you've heard a confusing list of good and bad fats to screen our menus and shopping lists for, but to keep things simple unprocessed fats are the good guys, while those which have been man-made are less so. Eggs, fish, nuts, seeds, liquid oils and avocado are all unprocessed natural sources of good, healthy fats and also loaded in vitamins. Margarine, cheese, processed oils (including coconut), baked goods such as cookies and croissants, and processed meats all contain trans fats that our body doesn't need and will struggle to process.

It is best to avoid these – as much as your tired, hungry body tells you 'fast food' is the way to go, it will give you little to nothing of what you need. If you can, avoid the pastries and make these your go-to 'fast foods': a boiled egg, a handful of nuts, a pot of yogurt or even a glass of milk.

Fill up on fibre

A balanced diet also needs to include a big dose of fibre, another hard to find essential in one-handed grabbed snacks and meals. Fibre is important to prevent a bloated, painful, gas-filled tummy and constipation, both of which we want to avoid like the plague! It's not only birth injuries that will thank you for keeping your bowel movements fluid, but your entire pelvic health. Avoiding constipation is a rule not just for the post-partum period, but for life. Constipation can lead to pelvic organ prolapse, haemorrhoids (blood vessels popping out of our bum), anal fissures (tears of the anus), pain and so on. And by constipation I don't just mean straining to pop out your number two, but not having a regular daily (at least once per day) bowel movement that is soft and easy to pass. A stool sitting within the rectum can weigh heavy on our pelvic floor, stretching the back wall of our vagina, which can lead to the posterior wall prolapsing into the vaginal space. The longer the stool sits there the more fluid is absorbed, making the stool firmer, harder to pass and potentially damaging the delicate anal tissue when it does finally exit.

We need our body's waste products to move through our gut and out quickly and efficiently, preventing stagnation, toxins being absorbed and our tissues becoming irritated. Many of us think of constipation as having to strain until we are red in the face, but this is only one sign that our stools are getting 'backed up'. Us women's health physios will often ask you what your poo looks like, which can be hard to explain! Fortunately, chocolate bars are universally recognisable, so I often use these to describe poo shape and consistency. It also sounds much more pleasant. If you're pooing formed, soft stools that look like a rippled Mars Bar then keep doing what you're doing. This is exactly what you want to see. If yours looks more like Maltesers or a few Maltesers squished together you probably don't need me to tell you that these are hard and difficult to pass. This can be a sign of constipation and the first change to make is to add more water to your day. If yours is more the opposite and coming out like chocolate sauce then fibre may be the missing ingredient in your diet. Follow my top tips for a daily habit to get yourself into the Mars Bar category!

- Drink more water. This is my go-to answer for a lot of things, but especially constipation. You need your stools to be soft enough to pass, the gut to be 'lubricated' and the bowel muscles to be well hydrated. Taking in excess water that you can afford to excrete is essential for this. If you are already drinking the recommended 1.5 litres a day, try adding just one more glass. If you're not getting close to this volume, you know what to do.

- If you're breastfeeding, first work out how much fluid your baby is taking from you. This is easy when you read the back of a pack of formula next time you're in the supermarket. For example, if it recommends that a baby the same age as yours should take five 150ml bottles a day, you know that you need to drink 750ml of water to feed your baby before your body will get any. Your gut needs to be well-hydrated to function and your stools need to be moist enough to move through your gut with ease to avoid associated problems. Enough said, so go grab yourself a healing glass of water!

- Check you're eating enough fibre. I'm sure you've heard 'eat more fibre' as the go-to cure for constipation. This is because it moves through the intestines undigested, adding bulk to the stool and encouraging regularity of bowel movements. Even if you think you are getting enough, try adding one of these foods to your daily diet and see how you feel? Our body's requirements change all the time, so perhaps you need a little more fibre now than you did last month. My favourite high fibre foods are:
  - Chia seeds, oat bran and flax seeds – just add a scoop to your cereal, on top of eggs, to soups, smoothies, pasta sauces…

- Legumes – essentially edible plants, including chickpeas, lentils, peas and peanuts.
- Berries, all of them – you can get great frozen selections so even when the fresh ones run out, you can stay topped up from the freezer.
- Kiwi fruit, apples and figs.

- Have a glass of prune or pear juice daily. These fruits contain magical sorbitol which draws water into the intestine, getting things moving.

- Take a dose of high magnesium leafy greens like kale and spinach or try a magnesium supplement. This is the main ingredient in many types of laxatives since it helps draw water into the intestines, encouraging things to pass through and out.

- To get things moving, get moving. When my babies were constipated, I remember learning techniques to help relieve them – pushing their legs to their chest and rolling their hips from side to side as well as massaging their swollen bellies in circles. It's no surprise that the same works for us too. A gentle walk and being up against gravity can also be very beneficial too.

- When going for a poo, pop your feet up on your kids' stool or invest in a Squatty Potty. This makes the angle of your rectum better positioned for gravity to assist your stool to drop down and out more easily. This is an absolute must to try before you even consider straining. If you are feeling tense it is likely your pelvic floor is too. Propping your feet up so that your knees are higher than your hips stretches your pelvic floor and helps it to relax and release. For a long time I kidded myself that leaning forwards worked just as well, but it really doesn't. Your knees higher than your hips is the key to a successful poo.

- Take probiotics to enhance your gut's beneficial bacteria and help out your digestive tract. The added bonus is that they are also good for immunity and heart health.

- De-stress, get pain free, carve out some time. If you're tense, in pain or rushing then your stools can happily (or rather unhappily) sit in the bowel paralysed. The tight tense, protective muscle spasm around the anus and pelvic floor can prevent the stool from dropping into the exit hatch. If you're struggling to relax on the loo, a women's health physiotherapist can help to manually release any tight and tense muscles which may be contributing to the toilet trouble. If you find that this is a continuous cycle then we can teach you how to manually release pelvic floor trigger points yourself. There are some great pelvic wands (they are magic!) that we can teach you to use to make this super-simple too.

Most of the time just a few small changes can make a huge difference. If you struggle to control your bowel movements with diet alone do visit your GP for a solution, such as a gentle laxative to get things moving, because when it comes to the consequences, prevention is better than cure.

I get it. You have enough on your plate (not literally) with a new baby and their routine, and your dietary needs are low on your list of priorities, but your baby needs you to bump it to the top, not just if you are breastfeeding and passing all that you eat directly to them, but also by demonstrating a healthy lifestyle and mindset on nutrition. The process of re-fuelling can be a real joy. Plan and prepare to avoid worry, stress or symptoms, and ask for help from family and friends.

Kimberly Ann Johnson's book: *The Fourth Trimester* is wonderful. I've shared her words with my family and would like to share them with you. Kimberly recommends new mothers find themselves a beautiful plate that speaks to them, that makes them smile, so that every meal feels like a gift and something to be cherished. This plate is just for them and should be presented at every mealtime as though it and the food it contains is a gift back to the mother. I think this is a rule we should all live by, whether woman or not, mother or child. Each meal we are fortunate to have is a gift and we each are a gift to each other. Since reading Kimberly's book I have been gathering a selection of wonderfully individual plates to fill our cupboards, so that every plate we eat from is special and everybody gets one.

TASK 17 SUPERCHARGED SNACKS

Smoothies and shakes have been a feature of most of my working life. They're the perfect snack to keep me going between clients in clinic and to boost my energy before and even while teaching. They really came into their own when I was pregnant with severe morning sickness, as the slow release got me through the nausea and sometimes even warded off the vomiting! As a new mum they were perfect for the time-poor, sleep-deprived me who needed to grab a quick something. The sweet hit from the fruit and protein kept me away from the cake cupboard and consequently the short-lived boost and post-energy slump that normally comes with high-sugar snacks. And I was happy to get my fruit and veggies in without having to pick up a knife and fork.

Tick everything off of your must-have checklist with this flexible, easy smoothie recipe. This is my favourite mix, but try your own too with the substitutions.

Protein: 1 scoop of KIN Vanilla No-Whey Pea protein. This tastes delicious and makes everything creamy and thick. They do a delicious dark chocolate one too. Vitimum (vitimum.com) is also great if you're expecting or breastfeeding as it packs all your essential vitamins in.

Leafy greens: 1 handful of frozen spinach. Frozen is key here, because there's nothing like a warm shake to make you gag! Kale, chard and bok choi work well too as you get all the green goodness without a strong taste.

Fibre: 1 tablespoon of flax seeds. These are great for regularity, and taste lovely and nutty, but chia seeds or oat bran work well too.

Sorbitol: half a pear. This sweetens things up, as well as giving us what we need for regular bowel movements. Sometimes I change this up for three prunes, a few dried apricots or figs with the same tastiness and effect.

Fats: 1 nice big spoon of peanut or almond butter. For a nut-free version, sub in coconut, avocado or whole yoghurt.

Water: A big cup-full to tick one off your list. No subs on this one I'm afraid!

Method: Mix it all up in a blender and enjoy.

I almost got through this section without mentioning weight loss. While maintaining a healthy weight is important for all our bodily functions, it is not the only reason we must consider what we feed our bodies. These engines of ours need the best fuel to run at their fullest potential, and this is never truer than in pregnancy and after birth.

When to ask for help:

- You are unable to open your bowels daily without straining.
- Your poo is always hard, pebble-like and difficult to pass.
- There is blood on the tissue when you wipe your bottom or pain when you poo. This could be an indication of a tear of your anus, which is called an anal fissure, but it can also be an indication of something more serious so please tell your GP.
- You have regular tummy pain and bloating that does not respond to the points outlined here.

What to ask for:

- When you have tried all of my tips for avoiding constipation your body may need an aid to make your daily habit more comfortable. Stool softener such as Dulcosoft or Movicol, which does as it says on the tin, makes poo softer and easier to pass. Or try a laxative such as Dulcolax or MiraLax, which works by stimulating the bowel muscles.
- Examination for an anal fissure and advice on healing this, because this will struggle to repair when the bowels are being opened and the injured tissue stretched on a daily basis, although it will heal when given the right care. An examination with your doctor and an accurate diagnosis is the first step towards this.
- Onward referral to a gastro-intestinal or colo-rectal specialist to further investigate changes with your dietary system that are not satisfactory.

What's important

- Drink water like a fish!
- Avoid constipation at all costs – address this early through diet and visit your GP for more support if you struggle to get this under control.

- Go for foods with slow-release energy to build the muscle you need to avoid energy negatives.
- Ensure you have enough protein for energy, healing and muscle growth.
- Fats are the building blocks of hormones and an essential part of our diet.
- Prepare meals and snacks when you have the time for when you don't. Call on your support network to help prepare, cook and/or deliver nutritious meals.

11. Sports and exercise: For body and mind

Being able to move our bodies is such a joy. Not being able to move them can be misery. As someone who works in fitness, being able to exercise without pain or discomfort is a must for me. For my body and mind, exercise is essential to keep me strong enough to work and play with my family, to keep me sane enough to tackle life and its everyday challenges, and to keep me connected to the friends I've met through a mutual love of exercise. As a physiotherapist my aim is always to help those with a goal to reach it – to break it down into achievable steps and address the weaknesses to make it possible.

We are all recommended to be physically active every day and spend at least 150 minutes a week on moderate intensity exercise, even in pregnancy, before even becoming pregnant and forever more. I know this sounds intimidating, but the benefits are vast and include reducing our risks of cardiovascular disease, diabetes, post-natal depression and even some cancers. Exercise serves as the best medicine in all these diseases, surpassing the benefits of drugs or other interventions. But you don't have to go to the gym every day or even start playing sport if this doesn't appeal to you. All sorts of exercise counts: a brisk walk on most days and a couple of Zoom exercise classes would be just fine.

The American College of Sports Medicine has outlined exactly what types of exercise are best and exactly what our ideal routine should entail:

- 30 minutes of cardiorespiratory exercise (exercise that makes you hot, sweaty and a little breathless) three to five times a week. This could include vigorous walking, jogging, swimming, cycling and so on.
- 30 minutes or more of strength training (that which makes your muscles ache) two to three times a week. While this includes lifting weights and resistance bands, your own body weight counts too. Classes such as Pilates,

body pump, legs, bums and tums, power yoga and body combat all come into this category.

- 20-30 minutes of stretching and balance training two to three times a week. This doesn't have to be yoga. You can work with any stretches. The important part is the stretches should be held for 30 seconds and repeated two to four times each. You can make up your own series from those you find in this book or follow a class online. Some classes you attend might also include a good stretch session, as well as a cardio or strength component.

These activities don't need to be taken on different days and some of my favourite classes include two or all of these components, like Pilates. Most Pilates classes last for 60 minutes and include strength, balance and stretching. HIIT (high intensity interval training) can also be incorporated into Pilates and then you can tick off all three goals: cardiovascular, strength and balance/stretch in just one class. I'm not just an advocate for Pilates classes either. There's circuit training, body balance, body pump, barre and many more that share these principles too. The important part is frequency. We should move our bodies daily to benefit our health in the physical and mental sense.

I understand that this can feel daunting and you are not alone. More than half of us aren't able to find the time and space to incorporate daily exercise and a quarter of us feel unable to exercise at all. There can be so many reasons that we may relate to for this, from lack of time, desire or childcare to not having the right space, support or kit to make this happen.

The power of exercise to heal a worried mind has been well-documented and it's recommended for stress, anxiety, depression and more. This is never truer than when you have recently given birth. Seeing your world and all it can hold through your baby's eyes is a real joy. Exercising alongside your baby, outdoors or at home is a stepping-stone for life and ignites the joy of movement, not just in us but in our children too. This was evident in the rise of the nation's PE teacher during the first 2020 lockdown. Joe Wicks engaged almost a million households, getting them to exercise together every weekday morning and starting a habit that I'm sure will last for years to come.

Our want, desire and motivation to engage in exercise often comes down to more than just knowing it's good for us. Understanding the health benefits is a factor, as well as perhaps finding the right social interaction. Walking with a friend, exercising in groups face to face or even virtually can be all we need to show up and move our bodies. It's totally OK to enjoy the social interaction more than the exercise – take from it what serves you and enjoy the health benefits. After both my babies were born I joined my local Buggyfit class (outdoor exercise for mums with babies in a buggy) as soon as they would have me. I longed to see other mums, chat and be outdoors, and the exercise was a bonus.

Whether you are new to regular exercise or it is a lifelong passion, please consider the following factors in getting there after pregnancy and birth.

When to start: It's not recommended you return to structured exercise regimes until six weeks post-partum. Before this time stick to your post-natal recovery as outlined in this book. From six weeks you can include more strength-based exercise, swimming and specialist post-natal exercise classes. Avoid anything impactful (running or jumping) for at least three months and ideally six.

Where to start: Swimming is great exercise for your pelvis, pelvic floor and abdominal recovery after birth. It works on those muscular slings which cross through your midline to give you the strength of guide ropes and tent pegs to keep your core strong. I don't recommend breast-stroke, which opens up the pelvis, but front crawl, back stroke and, my favourite; pull buoy. Swimming with a pull buoy is brilliant for the tummy, inner thigh and consequently the pelvic floor, because it acts just like the ball we have used in many of the exercises in tasks so far. Hold and squeeze the buoy between your legs while you pull through the water with your arms. It's my all-time favourite 'core' workout and is even great in pregnancy. Start with 20 minutes in the pool and slowly build on your time before increasing the intensity and speed.

Gym time: Cross training is another great cardiovascular workout that also strengthens the core, pelvic ring and all your muscular slings, as is uphill treadmill walking, especially if you work up to adding in hand weights. I recommend interval training for the best cardiovascular workout, which is also very time-efficient. You can work on interval goals of time or intensity. For example, work hard for 30 seconds at a high intensity, then rest and recover for 30 seconds at a lower intensity, repeating this for 20 minutes.

Load it up: Resistance-based training is beneficial not just for rehabilitation, but also injury prevention, health and wellbeing, bone density, boosting metabolism and weight loss. If you're not used to lifting weights (apart from babies and children!) a personal training session or body pump class would be a great place to start. Reformer Pilates is also a good example of resistance-based training and with Joseph Pilates' focus on the core it fits perfectly with rebuilding goals after pregnancy.

Take it down: Start with a lower intensity version of what you enjoy. If it's a 45-minute spin class, get back into it with 30-minute foundation classes to ensure you're ready. If it's competitive sport, aim for several weeks of training before you put yourself on the court, pitch or field. Lower the intensity, duration and speed of your exercise and slowly build it up again.

Fix your goal: Whatever your sport, this is your end goal not your starting point. Complete your pelvis, pelvic floor and abdominal rehabilitation as the first step in getting there. Next comes sport-specific strengthening. What does your body need to be able to do, repeatedly, in your sport? Break this down and practise this. Strengthen and condition your body to avoid injury and smoothly get back to what you enjoy.

Recovery times: Following a significant soft tissue injury, which, let's be honest, 'regular' childbirth counts as, you need to allow three months for complete rehabilitation. You may well return to sport or exercise within this time, but it has to be a progressive return alongside strengthening. Therefore, following 'natural' birth you should allow *at least* three months before returning to running, impact exercise, contact and explosive sports (any which involve sudden movement). Now if there has been a separation of the muscle, a tear or a cut (as in a Caesarean or episiotomy), you need the tissues to not only heal but repair stronger than they were before. It then takes a further three months of progressive loading to grow a bigger muscle. Add this up and you are looking at six months of rehabilitation and strengthening before returning to high-impact exercise after vaginal birth with trauma or an abdominal birth. Some will feel strong enough before this milestone, some will take longer. Use this as a gentle guide to give yourself time and space to protect, stabilise and rehabilitate.

You might think walking is the obvious starting point, but walking after pregnancy and birth needs to be considered as exercise like any other. Walking is an essential part of our everyday lives, but can pose a real challenge to healing and recovery after pregnancy and birth. When we walk one foot leaves the ground, putting 100% of our body weight on the opposite leg and pelvis. The muscles here, and through our pelvic floor and waist, have to work harder to stabilise while the other leg swings through. The contraction and strength needs to quickly switch sides before the next step. If we don't have enough stability through our pelvic ring and abdominal cylinder we can stress and strain its joints and muscles and potentially destabilise our post-natal pelvis and pelvic floor further.

So although it is often considered the starting point for exercise after birth, walking can actually be quite a challenge for a post-partum body. While it is important to walk, and I am certainly not banning this activity altogether, I recommend limiting it to a maximum of 30 to 60 minutes a day in your first six weeks following pregnancy and birth. You must increase your strength before progressing to longer walks as these will provide your body with the protection and stability it needs to prevent destabilising your pelvis and pelvic floor when walking.

The return to running after pregnancy and birth has been given much attention and thankfully there are now specific return-to-run criteria, but it is not just running that you need to prepare your body and rebuild your strength for post-partum. Mountain biking, tennis, racquet ball and contact sports, skiing and many more besides all give the body impactful and explosive challenges that our muscles, joints and organs need to be stable and strong enough to withstand. In preparation for return to running or any sport you need to ensure you are strong enough and ready. Again, this starts with loaded strengthening in the most stable positions before you consider more dynamic challenges.

You can see a pattern here, huh?! Strength, strength, strength. It's an essential component to our health and wellness that is too often overlooked, not fully understood and reserved for gym-goers, but let me remind you that this book is called *Stronger*. It contains all you need to regain strength without ever having to step inside a gym.

TASK 18 A CORE WORKOUT

KIT YOU WILL NEED: A bench or sofa. Add hand weights or wear them in a backpack as your strength builds for a greater challenge.

This core workout circuit incorporates the muscle groups most challenged after pregnancy and birth – the ones you need to rebuild to return to sport. Weakness here can be responsible for pain, injury and dysfunction on return to activity. You're going to use the pain-free movements and automatic firing of your pelvic floor and tummy that you've ticked off in previous tasks, so you should be progressing to here rather than using this as your starting point.

Your goal is 4 minutes' work on each exercise, 20 working minutes in total. You can try 30 seconds of each x4, building up to 45 seconds and then 60 seconds as you feel stronger.

Calf raise hold:

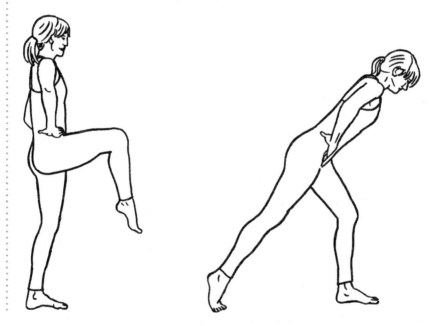

Calf raises are great for strength down your back line, tightening up your foot arches and bringing the weight away from the front of the knee where it can get sore. Stand on one leg with a soft bend in your knee, then lift your heel up and down for as long as you can, aiming for 30 seconds x3 on each side. See if you can add a fourth, fifth or even sixth set as your strength and endurance builds. Try and keep your pelvis level and your chest proud to keep your bottom active too.

Standing scooter/leg thruster: Start in a scooter position with one leg straight and out behind you, the other slightly bent and your body weight forwards. As you breathe out lift your back leg off the floor and up to your chest as you bring your body upright, then keep your balance as you take this leg back behind. Return to your start position. That's one rep! You're aiming for 10 in total followed by a 10-second hold. Repeat this twice with no rest, then change sides. This mimics the strength, balance and endurance you need on one leg for most sports. You can progress from here by increasing the number of sets from two to three then four, five and even six in a row with no rest. Feel the burn!

Hip bridge marches: Shoulder bridge for strength in your back and bottom with your shoulders rested on a sofa edge or chair. From here, keep your pelvis dead level and raise one leg. Alternate your legs so that you are marching. The important part is to keep your bottom high and level, and feel the work in the grounded leg. Aim for one continuous minute of marching, followed by 15 seconds' rest, and repeat three times. You can add a fourth and fifth set as you improve.

Adductor plank leg lifts: Adductor plank is my all-time favourite measure of return-to-run strength. You weight-bear on the inside thigh of the top leg and the bottom arm and waist. The force crosses at your midline bringing strength to your centre. Start with a short lever, a bent top leg, rested on a chair and put the bottom leg on the ground to share a little bit of the load if you need to. When you can hold this for 30 seconds, change sides. Do three sets. For an extra challenge lift and lower the bottom leg as you hold your plank and form. As your strength builds you can start to straighten your top leg and move further away from the chair so that your shin is bearing your weight, then further still so that you have a straight top leg with your weight going through your foot – just as in running (you can see an illustration of this exercise on page 146).

Rotating side plank:

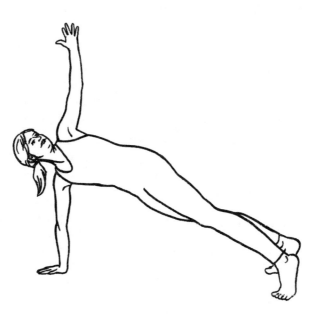

Start in your plank position with your hands underneath your shoulders, arms straight, and your feet hip-width apart. Keep your spine in neutral as you rotate to one side, lifting one hand to the sky, and roll to the borders of your feet for side plank. Pause here before rolling back to plank, then rotate to the other side. Aim for 30 secs with great form x4 sets with 15 seconds rest between then. You can build your endurance to 45 seconds and then 60 seconds.

I am often asked if we should be consciously contracting the pelvic floor while running or playing sport. The simple answer is no. The long-winded version is absolutely not, because you will overwork your pelvic floor, undoubtedly change your normal running style or movement patterning, risking injury, and likely take all the fun out of what you previously enjoyed. Much like training for any event, rebuilding after pregnancy and birth is a process and once you have rebuilt your strength and stability you will have gained enough for your sport. If you leak, feel pain or prolapse in your sport then you are not yet ready, and need to continue to rehabilitate to build up to the level of strength you need. Instead, incorporate your pelvic floor and tummy tension exercises in the task above to build the strength you need.

This is not to say you should never contract your pelvic floor in sport or exercise, but rather that you should only do it when you need it. For example, if you're returning to tennis you may start to train hitting a ball with your outbreath, which will encourage an upward movement of your pelvic floor, rather than holding your breath, which would increase the load and pressure. You can also minimise the load, pressure and impact on the joints and muscles of your abdominal cylinder and pelvic ring with a few other considerations:

Footwear: A great time to invest in new sports shoes is after having a baby. Your shape, strength and stability has undoubtedly changed. You may need more support and cushioning now where you didn't before. New shoes will always provide more cushioning than old ones, meaning less impact further up your pelvic ring and abdomen.

Keep it steady: Uneven surfaces will require a greater and more explosive and responsive strength than consistent and steady movement patterning. Run on even ground, ski the easy runs and play on sand-less courts.

Reduce the impact: Harder surfaces, jumps and bumps, and running downhill will all increase the force going up through your body. Minimise this by playing, training and running on softer (but stable) ground. Avoid impact or contact sports and walk down hills while embracing the uphill climbs and flats.

Pregnancy and motherhood are times of huge physical and psychological change and adjustments to our normal exercise regime is part of this. We can embrace these changes and opportunities to try something new, and to choose to engage in exercise that fits our body's needs is a real strength. Try not to feel restricted by what does not suit you or feel good right now – the post-natal period is a time to get comfortable with a lower intensity and level of exercise. Embrace this recovery period and set realistic goals. You may well then over-achieve, over-accomplish and surprise yourself.

When to ask for help:

- If you leak urine when you run or play sport. Despite what you might hear it is not normal to have to wear a pad to exercise. This is a sign that your body cannot yet take the pressures of running or playing and you need to protect, stabilise and rehabilitate. Tick off all you can from the tasks in this book and if you still have symptoms please seek help and treatment.

- You have joint pain that stops you from engaging in activities you enjoy.

- Your energy or mood is too low to move from your sofa, let alone exercise.

What to ask for:

- A physiotherapy or women's health referral to teach you exactly what, where and how to strengthen your body for your goals, although you might have to pay for this it will be worth it.

- You can also enlist the support of a personal trainer or exercise specialist, but this would be a personal expense.

- Blood tests to check for hormonal abnormalities, which could be depleting your energy and good mood.

- Mental health support – this could be as simple as a friendly face and a chat with your doctor, but there is a whole range of support out there if you are struggling with anxiety, depression or negativity towards your body and what it can do now. You've just got to speak up and trust there is *never* judgement.

What's important

- It is not recommended to return to structured physical exercise before six weeks after giving birth (this does not include prescriptive healing and rebuilding exercises, and definitely excludes pelvic floor exercises, which you can start from day one).

- Impact exercise is not recommended before a minimum of three months post-partum. No negotiations. After surgical birth or birth injury six months is a minimum time frame for return to impact sports and explosive exercises in order to protect your healing body. If you feel ready before this, I encourage you to visit a women's health physiotherapist who can give you the OK.

- Return to impact exercise should be progressive, meaning little by little not all at once, from three months after birth at the earliest, but it may be better if you can give your body a full 6 months to heal.

- Whatever your goal, break it down and work on the strength needed to make it more achievable, and to minimise risk of injury and pelvic floor symptoms.

- Every woman should aim to move their body every day and spend at least 150 minutes a week on moderate intensity exercise for maximum health benefits. If your body holds you back from achieving this, please ask for help and support to get there.

12. Intimacy: Pleasure, connection and sex

Sexual desires, pleasure, wants, needs and enjoyment all are closely related to how our body is feeling. Feeling pain free, proud of our bodies, strong and capable, being able to move, engage, and enjoy are all givens until they are not. Getting back there is part of your recovery and this journey to heal and rebuild. While I am far from a 'sexpert', I recognise that the issues we have addressed so far can also have an impact on our sexual relationships. The most common questions I get asked about sex after pregnancy and birth are 'When is it OK?' and 'Will it cause me any damage?'.

When is it OK?

When you, your body and your partner feel ready. That's it. The only word of caution is if there are healing wounds or scars to your tummy, vagina, perineum or back passage. Then I recommend refraining from sex in all forms for a minimum of four to six weeks or until they have healed. If you have experienced these injuries then this advice may feel obvious and sex is likely the last thing you want to consider, but just in case! You want to avoid infection by touching or inserting anything around there, keep your healing tissues as still as possible to encourage them to knit back together and to prevent re-stretching these delicate parts. Four to six weeks is the standard time for wounds to heal and toughen up, *unless* there has been an infection or re-opening. In which case be guided by your GP or the midwife who will be reviewing your healing and don't be embarrassed to ask directly if and when sex will be OK given you are slightly off course from these average healing times.

Aside from this, there is no set amount of time for which you should refrain from sex after birth. Equally there is no time by which you *should* have had sex following birth. We heal at different rates and recovery from birth is needed before we can feel ready to have sex again. When I mention sex in my post-natal MOTs most women tell me with a shy giggle that they have not even contemplated the act since their little one's arrival. Lack of sleep, sharing your bedroom with your baby, the rollercoaster of emotions and exhaustion are unlikely to put you in the mood for sex, making love or even a 'quickie'. I get it, of course. I felt the same way, but I always follow up by asking if it's something they're worried about, afraid of or avoiding for any reason. Most admit that they're not feeling very sexy right now and I want to give them all a big hug, which I sometimes do (or did pre-Covid!). As part of their MOT I offer them an examination to check that they have fully healed, assess what feels painful, gauge how much stretch their new tissues can tolerate and ultimately reassure them. You can do this yourself. I get you're not a physio or an anatomy expert, but you are the best judge of what feels nice, safe and enjoyable. I will show you how in task 19.

Will it cause me any damage?

I recommend using pain as your guide on this one. Generally speaking, post-partum sex should not cause harm or any pain (after your initial four to six week recovery period if there has been any trauma). Pain is our body's way of protecting us, a warning sign to avoid harm. If you experience any pain with physical touch or penetrative sex I recommend stepping back from this and sticking to only what feels good. Don't lean into the pain, but work around it – your body will heal and you'll feel ready to go further when it does.

Surprisingly, something I am rarely asked is how to start. Now this is probably the last thing grown women want to ask me, their physiotherapist, but to me it seems comfortable and normal to discuss this, like any other rehabilitation goal. However, to avoid the embarrassment I've written it all down so you can read it when you're ready.

Position of the fortnight – anyone else remember this highlight from now defunct teen magazine *More!*? Don't you think it would have been helpful to include some sexual position guidelines with our pregnancy folder alongside those flyers for nappies and pads? How exactly to get comfortable and orgasm when we have a big bump and a baby sitting on-top of our bladder, haemorrhoids plaguing our bottom and our vagina swelling unrecognisably would have been really helpful! And what about now, after birth?

Finding out right now what positions are best considering your unique birth and recovery will answer many unasked questions I'm sure. Questions like: 'Is missionary OK with a Caesarean scar?', 'Can I straddle if I've had a perineal tear?' or 'How do I have an active sex life with back pain after pregnancy?' So here they are, *my positions of the *fortnight* (* by fortnight I mean can last you as long as you like!)

Missionary: Partner on top, you're underneath, legs akimbo.

Do it: If you had any cuts or tears to your vagina or perineum this is a good position in which to test out penetration. You are face to face with your partner and can feed back directly how good or bad things feel and anything you are nervous or scared of. You can figure it out together by watching each other's expressions. Your partner also can't go as deep into your vagina here (providing you keep your legs on the bed and not wrapped around their head!) which can be reassuring the first few times you 'do it'.

Don't do it: This is not so good if you have back or pelvic pain as you have to carry your partner's weight on top of your pelvis, which can be uncomfortable. Also, it's not great if your tummy scar is still healing after an abdominal birth.

Spoon: Where you're both lying on your side, you in front and facing away with penetration from behind.

Do it: This is great if you've had an abdominal birth as your tummy is relaxed and out of the 'thrusting' zone. It's also a great one if you are conscious at all of your tummy shape after pregnancy. The last thing you want right now is body hang-ups and I assure you your bottom looks great from where your partner is! I also recommend this if you've been having back or pelvic pain, but you'll need to try and rest your top leg on a pillow rather than lifted to keep your pelvis comfortable.

Don't do it: If you've had a perineal tear of any degree or an episiotomy it's likely going to kill the moment if your partner slips and you're jabbed where your scars lie in the perineum or anus.

Cowgirl: You sit on top and straddle your partner, like riding a horse. Penetration can be deep here, but you are in control.

Do it: This can be a great position if you have had any birth injuries, including cuts, tears, back or pelvic pain and abdominal birth scars. You are in control and both yours and your partners hands are free for more fun. You can easily climb down for oral pleasure if you're not quite feeling penetration and, again, you can feed back to one another with expression as you're face to face.

Don't do it: You look gorgeous from up there, trust me. There's no reason not to try this one, but you might want to save it for when you are a little less knackered and can give it some welly!

Doggy-style: Animalistic and oh so good for both of you as you share the control. You're on all fours, or elbows and knees, and penetration is from behind with your partner kneeling or standing.

Do it: If you have back or pelvic pain this is a great rehab position, so you can tick off some of your day's strengthening exercise while also getting a good sex session in! This position is also good for your tummy if you have a healing scar as there's no friction and you can relax it. Confidence-boosting as you look great and you can add in clitoral stimulation with hands and toys as much as you desire.

Don't do it: Things are going deep here so if you're sore at all on the inside it's best to put this one on the back burner for a little while. Also, if you had cuts or tears to your vagina or perineum there can be a big old stretch to them here, which is safe and likely won't harm you, but may sting a little and feel stretchy to start with.

It's important to highlight here how many forms of sex we can enjoy. Often we think of penetrative sex as the only sex, the pinnacle or end goal. 'Everything but' is deemed as not quite there, but how rubbish is that? I for one get just as much enjoyment from 'everything but' and I know that I am not the only one – 78% of women will not climax with penetrative sex alone and need clitoral stimulation to reach the big O. Shockingly, one sex study found that 100% of men climax from penis in vagina sex, compared to 10% of women. This is not acceptable. Sex is not a luxury to be enjoyed by only one half of the party. If the idea of penetrative sex is scary or off-putting for you don't let this put you off the idea of intimacy altogether. It is not the only way you can share this closeness again.

Often when discussing a return to sexual intimacy women say to me 'My poor partner…' or 'My partner is chomping at the bit'. I want to shout, 'What about *you*?' In pregnancy and birth our vaginas become 'the birth canal', a medicalised passage for examinations, midwife's fingers and what sometimes feels like the whole world to look at, but we are much more than our vaginas. The rest of our sexual selves has not been medicalised. No one other than our partner has seen us become putty in their hands as they touch all the right buttons and arouse us with kisses and whole-body intimacy. If, like most women, you orgasm from clitoral stimulation then leave your vagina out of this for as long as you can. Get back to your sexual self without those reminders of your recent experiences and in time you can reclaim your vagina's sexual identity.

Protect

You can protect your healing self and prevent any risk of infection in wounds or your settling womb by not allowing anything inside or around your vagina for the first four to six weeks, but clitoral stimulation is very OK. Thankfully your clitoris is far enough away from your vagina and the opposite side to your perineum (where most birth scars are likely to be). Your 'clit' is positioned on the outside of your body just below the top fold of your labia, so massaging, flicking, licking and vibeing here are all totally fine.

After pregnancy and birth lubrication is an essential part of sexual pleasure and, when you are ready, intercourse. This is even more so if you are breastfeeding as the hormonal changes that come with pregnancy, birth and lactation can play havoc with your vagina's natural lubrication. As a result, you may experience vaginal discomfort, burning, itching or pain, not just during and after sex but day to day, making it much less likely that you feel 'up for it' in the first place. You can compensate for this with natural and PH-balanced personal lubricants to not only soothe, heal and nourish sensitive tissues, but also to ease painful sex and provide glide over friction. And don't just save these for the bedroom. There are many lubricants that can also be used as vaginal moisturisers. Think how your facial skin care regime has changed since your teenage years, through adult life and pregnancy to now. You may need to support your body's, and particularly your vagina's, response to hormonal changes just as you do with your skincare regime. A daily soothing lubricant such as those by

YesYesYes could be just what you need to relive pain, restore comfort and boost your libido.

Stabilise

Intimate touch, orgasms and early pelvic floor exercises will help to heal and rebuild your nerves and the muscles. Think of it as a re-education. Sending signals along the nerve-to-muscle pathway to contract, tighten, release and let go will improve the blood flow, healing and also your body's ability to become aroused.

For those with birth injuries I recommend starting your perineal scar massage as soon as there is adequate tissue healing, (see task 6 on page 83, but just to recap that's only from four to six weeks when the wound has fully closed and there's no weeping or stitches left). Perineal scars can feel tight and raw, making penetrative sex uncomfortable and sometimes painful. Scar massage with your hands or a vibrator is a great way to moisturise, mobilise and prepare these tissues for the natural stretch and sensation of intercourse. You can even ask your partner to help. Who knows, you may even start to enjoy it!

When returning to sexual activity with your partner I 100% recommend declaring a period of 'extended foreplay' or sex without penetration. If you jump into bed with both you and your partner knowing that penetrative sex is off the table it is likely you will both feel more relaxed, comfortable to explore, share and enjoy your post-partum body. Receiving and giving sexual pleasure without penetration can be hugely beneficial to your physical and emotional recovery. I'm sure your partner will gladly receive this information and participate enthusiastically in this leg of your rehab journey.

Rehabilitate

Let this become the easiest task in this book! We can approach healing and rebuilding our sexual selves just like any other body part or function. Break the challenge down so that it is achievable and then add in some task-specific training. Sounds fun, huh?

Getting to know how your vagina, perineum and pelvic floor feel before anyone else does is the first step towards your end goal. As I've already mentioned, clitoral stimulation and orgasm are brilliant for pelvic floor, vaginal and perineal scar healing. Sexual excitation and climax engorge your vagina and ultimately your pelvic floor with blood, which is perfect when you want to heal injured tissues. An orgasm elicits a series of powerful contractions of your vaginal and pelvic floor muscles, so instead of more conscious squeezing and releasing you are going to work towards these involuntary excitations instead. And you thought doing your pelvic floor exercises was dull!

TASK 19 NAVIGATING THE NETHER REGIONS

Please don't wait until you have worked through the rest of my book to try this! You can enjoy this task anytime and it may even enhance your success with the others.

KIT YOU WILL NEED: A map and compass (just kidding), a quiet place where you feel safe and relaxed, and a natural, silky lube, balm or oil.

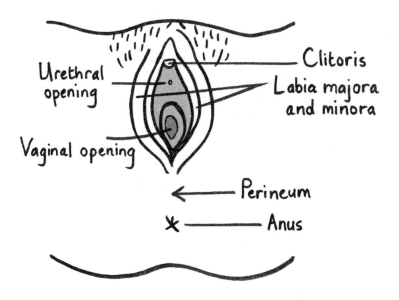

You may want to use a mirror so you know where you're going, but the most important thing you'll need is comfort. The bath is a great place to do this as your body and hands will be warm or on your bed with a luscious balm and warm hands is just as good. If you are worried about pain or discomfort a small vibrator is a good way to overcome this. Vibration is a tool we use often to de-sensitise – when the body feels vibration it overpowers the detection of pain and it feels pretty awesome too.

Your main objective is to work out what feels good and what doesn't. To better get to know and be comfortable with your post-baby body, start at your tummy. Rub in circles or trace the vibrator around in a clockwise direction below your tummy button. This can be a super-sensitive, often uncomfortable and sometimes numb area post-birth, especially following abdominal birth. Gentle touch from your partner here can go one of two ways, so it's good to be comfortable with your own touch first. What pressure on your tummy is comfortable? Can you tolerate firmness or just the lightest of touches? This will help you figure out what sexual positions you might feel most comfortable with.

After a few minutes here move on to your inner thighs. Massage again with your hands or a vibrator from mid-thigh all the way up to your pubic arch, where your legs meet in the middle. Is it uncomfortable to open your legs? If so, work on one at a time. This can be painful if you suffered with back or pelvic pain, so take it slowly if you anticipate this. Again, you are working out what you are comfortable with so change position to your side if this feels better for you.

Moving on after several minutes to your labia, lightly trace down one side, across your perineum, move up the other side and cross the top above your clitoris. If that's comfortable increase your pressure, change direction or your touch. If your birth involved cuts, tears or intervention this can feel scary as the last person touching you down there was a doctor, so take your time. Stop here if you need to and come back to this task another day. A nourishing balm should feel great on your skin. Ice and warm oils are also good to try, especially if your sensation is reduced.

And then you can move on to your clitoris. Remember your task is to find what feels good, either just for you or so that you can share this information with your partner and return to intimacy. A lot of sensation may be overwhelming, so again go slowly. What feels good here? A light touch? More pressure? Vibration? Explore and relax. Your post-partum body is a miracle and one to be enjoyed.

Finally, and if you want to, explore around your vaginal opening and inside your body. Map out erogenous zones. Do you have a G-spot? Does this feel nice or are you keen to get back to your clit? Is there anything here that is painful or strange for you to touch? Only when this feels OK would you want to think about penetrative sex, but look at all you've crossed to get here and remember that the end goal is your pleasure, not just penetration.

If sex in any form is your last remaining goal and you want to know more I cannot recommend enough the Hot Bed Collective. Their hugely helpful and positive book and podcasts are the perfect tools. Let's not ignore this piece of the puzzle and important step in rebuilding you.

When to ask for help:

- If sex is painful or causes distress or bleeding.
- You feel anxious, scared or worried about returning to intimacy.
- Despite saying no, you experience unwanted sexual pressure, advances or touch.

What to ask for:

- A gynaecological review to assess your healing vaginal and perineal tissues. If needed, further treatment or physiotherapy may then be recommended.
- Counselling for psychological birth trauma, sexual exploration or marital support. This may need to be self-funded, but your doctor can point you in the right direction and offer a friendly ear.

What's important

- Sexual pleasure and climax are good for your recovery (have I mentioned that yet?!). Start with clitoral stimulation. Take intercourse off the table and make pleasure your goal.
- If sexual intercourse is your goal, break it down into achievable steps like any other challenge.
- Start your perineal massage and pelvic floor exercises as soon as you can to return normal vaginal, perineal and pelvic floor sensations.
- Orgasms are great.

13. Hormones: The good, the bad and the monthly

When it comes to feeling stronger, we must now also consider the very building blocks of our being. Hormones often get a bad rap, but they are essential for, well, everything! They are chemical messengers for every bodily movement, function and reaction, and not just responsible for 'mood swings'. Hormones are powerful creatures and even the slightest rise or fall in their levels can lead to huge changes within our bodies. This is never more so than in pregnancy and the post-natal period. Most of the time we are blissfully unaware of our hormones and their magic actions and interactions within us, there are over 50 different types made by the human body. Yep, that's right – men have hormones too. There may be a few that you already know, are household names and you frequently pull your hair out over, but it may surprise you to know that these hormones are not just made by women. So here are some truths about 'women's hormones'.

Follicle stimulating hormone (FSH): This is involved in the menstrual cycle in women, but did you know it is also made by men and essential for making sperm?

Luteinizing hormone (LH): Working with FSH, this makes us ovulate. In fellas, LH is also present, stimulating sperm production and raising testosterone.

Oxytocin: Not just present to form bonds between mother and baby and father and baby, oxytocin is also involved in sexual arousal and is produced with orgasms. This gives both men and women an emotional bond with the orgasm-maker!

Sex hormones: As oestrogen and progesterone, known as the 'female sex hormones', and testosterone, known as the 'male sex hormone', are present in both sexes technically they're really just 'sex hormones'. They are responsible for the development of our sex organs, arousal and reproduction. Amazingly when we ovulate around our male partners their testosterone spikes, apparently subconsciously detecting the changes in our 'scent', making the chances of sex much more likely! These sex hormones and their balance together are integral to the miracle of pregnancy.

Prolactin: This is involved in making breast milk and the changes to our breasts which enable us to feed our babies, but it is also produced by guys and girls during orgasm and makes our bits spasm with excitement. Cool huh!

Our hormones often come faced with a lot of criticism when, in fact, they deserve some respect for all the awesome things they do. The human body is amazing.

We cannot always predict what our hormones are up to, especially after having a baby, when we are breast feeding or have hormonal birth control (if that's our choice – it's not everyone's). Often our six-week check-up is an opportunity to discuss birth control measures with our doctor and you may well have already restarted with your preferred method, be it pill, coil, implant or another approach, but it's still worth knowing what is naturally occurring within our bodies and recognising the changes, whether our cycle is medically controlled or otherwise.

Progesterone is an essential hormone in becoming pregnant and is often blamed or given credit for early hormonal changes such as bigger breasts and morning sickness. Progesterone is also a smooth muscle relaxant, which allows our uterus to stretch and accommodate our growing baby. But, as with all hormones, it has an effect on all of our bodily functions and not just our uterus. The smooth muscles of our bladder, bowel and pelvic floor are also affected. Suddenly being able to hold a full bladder, fully empty our bowel or support our pelvic organs becomes much harder in pregnancy, even before our baby bump is visible. Shortly after birth our progesterone levels drop dramatically, but they will rise and fall again during our monthly cycles. Just before our period there is a sudden spike in this muscle-relaxing hormone, which is a time that many women report incontinence or urgency, and prolapse symptoms are often worse during this time of the month. As in pregnancy, the muscles of the pelvic floor, bladder and bowel become more relaxed as a result and so we need more strength just prior to and over the first few days of our period than at other times of the month.

The pelvic floor, bladder and urethra contain oestrogen receptors, so although we might not be aware of it, oestrogen helps to maintain tone and tension in these muscles all the time. This can balance out the progesterone effect in pregnancy when oestrogen levels are high, but it can be problematic when they drop suddenly after birth, during our monthly cycle or at menopause. Oestrogen levels can drop even further below our normal baseline when we are breastfeeding as high oestrogen interferes with milk production. Instead, prolactin, the hormone mostly responsible for milk production, kicks in.

Prolactin can have a knock-on effect on our happy hormone, dopamine. Dopamine gives us feelings of euphoria and happiness, which, as new mothers with our world in our arms, we probably have in abundance. But prolactin can hit dopamine levels hard and, together with less sleep than normal and a drop off in oestrogen, these euphoric feelings can be hard to find and they can be replaced by low energy levels, sudden and extreme highs and lows, and even a slower metabolism for many months after birth. Cue the 'baby blues'. Other mothers can often spot this in us as they remember it only too well, but in my experience, even though we have heard this phrase before, it can be hard to recognise this in ourselves.

We are often so underprepared for this sudden drop in mood – not helped by a lack of anything familiar to latch on to in this new life and identity as a mother. What we should, could or hoped to feel stirs up guilt and longing, instead of us just being kind and gentle with ourselves. It might be helpful to remind yourself that these times will pass, like a hunger or feeling tired. Your internal chemical matrix will rebalance and you will recognise yourself again soon enough. If you feel that your hormones have rebalanced, but the way you are feeling hasn't picked up, do seek some support. Don't feel embarrassed or ashamed – you need your cup filled before you can fill anyone else's. If you're going to care for another being, you first need to take care of yourself.

I remember one incredibly tough time in those newborn days, trying to explain to my husband that I didn't want the pain of trying to breastfeed and the frustration of failing again, nor for our daughter to be fed with a bottle. While she screamed in hunger I stood in the way of her getting the bottle in my husband's hands, while also protectively covering up my already leaking breasts. We were both at a loss of what to do and how to navigate these hormone-fuelled tides of determination, love and fear. We eventually settled for both. Our daughter hungrily filed her tummy with a small bottle then fed a little from me, with us both a little less desperate, less determined and less emotional. After my tears had passed and our daughter slept contentedly we laughed at this, and could both be kind and forgiving, and discuss a better plan for feeding ahead of next time.

It can take six to eight weeks after giving birth or stopping breastfeeding for your hormones to return to their normal balance. This means that if you feed for six months, a year or more, it can take a further six to eight weeks on top of this for your body to return to your hormonal 'normal'. Until then, physical and psychological changes as a result are to be expected. While we cannot change this, we can perhaps manage our own and others' expectations. Be patient, tolerant and kind to yourself, and those around you will be too.

But it is not just in the baby-making years that our hormonal changes can bring us unwanted symptoms. Symptoms due to hormonal changes that may arise cyclically as well as after pregnancy are:

- Constipation: The efficiency in the smooth muscles of our bowel is affected which can make bowel movements more irregular and harder to pass.

- Heaviness, discomfort and incontinence related to pelvic organ prolapse as strength, tone and holding capacity is down.

- Leaking urine, urgency or frequency in visiting the loo. Our bladder, bowel and pelvic floor may struggle to hold as much at certain times of the month as others.

- Pelvic, back and vaginal pain as a result of muscular cramps and tissue engorgement.

- Low mood or sudden changes in our feelings.

- Sleep disturbances.

Oestrogen levels dip twice every menstrual cycle; following ovulation and towards the end of our period, and of course at menopause. When our oestrogen levels drop so does the tone and tension in our essential pelvic floor muscles. If we are dependent on having oestrogen around for tone, our muscles may struggle at these times of the month or at menopause and symptoms will be more apparent. This is why pelvic floor dysfunction has historically been considered a feature of the menopausal years, something for older women to contend with, prepare for and even endure (repeat after me: 'Not I!').

These symptoms do not ever need to be features of our monthly cycle or life. If we have a greater amount of muscle tone and strength to start with, we can cope with the changes life brings us. The better our baseline strength then the less likely it is that a drop-off in tone as a result of hormonal changes will affect us. If we enter pregnancy, motherhood and menopause with a good, functioning, strong pelvic floor and stable pelvic ring then we can stay symptom free, despite the challenges these phases bring. Clients often tell me they are fine all month long until the start of their period. Their concern, and rightly so, is that this could be a sign of things to come with menopause. Sure, it's easy to ignore 'bladder weakness' on a few days a month, especially with the normalisation and accessibility of pads and sanitary products for just these occasions, but what if we take these days as warnings signs instead of something to be expected and put up with? Warning signs that our capacity is down, that we need more strength, that our muscle system is dependent on a fine line of hormonal balance to keep us dry and comfortable. We can wait and see, ignore the warning signs and easily forget until next month, but the sooner we act the more chance we have to raise our threshold, to increase the capacity of the pelvic floor and ultimately avoid symptoms. If we are strong enough most of the month, but challenged by hormonal changes at certain times, let's increase our strength so that even with peaks and troughs in hormone levels and muscle tone we stay above the symptom threshold and give ourselves the best chance of being able to ignore those bladder ads on TV.

What our body needs over the different stages of our menstrual cycle is as varied as how we feel over this time, both physically and mentally. You may have noticed this when instead of hitting the gym you just want to curl up on the sofa and then, unsurprisingly, your period arrives the next day. Or you've heard of the amazing phenomenon whereby women wear fewer clothes when they are ovulating as some sort of 'evolutionary call to procreate' (or maybe just because our body temperature sits a few degrees higher?!).

If we better understand what's heading our way hormonally then we can plan our activities and lives accordingly. And what if we sync our pelvic floor exercises with our cycle too and give our body exactly what it needs each week of the month to benefit from our cyclical energies?

TASK 20 HORMONE HARMONY

KIT YOU WILL NEED: A menstrual cycle, and task 3 and 4 (see pages 55–58) ticked off.

A quick note: this is not a starting point for healing and rebuilding, but more of a final progression. Once you have healed and recovered your strength by working through the preceding chapters, only then take on this mastery of synchronising your pelvic floor exercise with your monthly cycle.

Once you've restored your pelvic floor strength, pelvic function and tummy tone you need to keep things ticking along with a maintenance programme, but even I as a physiotherapist get bored of the same rehabilitation exercises. It's always tempting to try something new, something out of your routine that

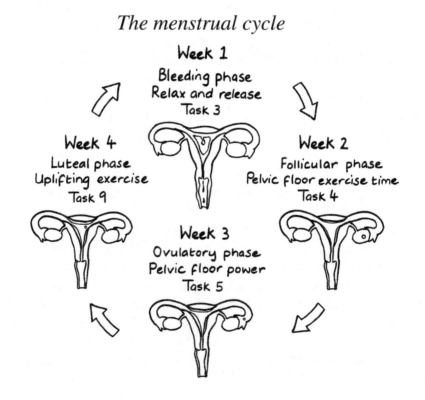

The menstrual cycle

Week 1
Bleeding phase
Relax and release
Task 3

Week 4
Luteal phase
Uplifting exercise
Task 9

Week 2
Follicular phase
Pelvic floor exercise time
Task 4

Week 3
Ovulatory phase
Pelvic floor power
Task 5

you've not built up to, but before you know it you're in that trampoline class and, oops, back to square one! To keep on track with pelvic floor exercises for life (or at least up until menopause when they will change again) I recommend mixing your pelvic floor rehabilitation up throughout the month. Change your exercises on a weekly basis in balance with your body and to avoid boredom and repetition.

Week 1 – bleeding phase: Energy is at its lowest this week so choose exercise and activities which reflect this. Work on both contracting and fully relaxing your pelvic floor to release tense muscles and ease discomfort.

Review task 3 on page 55. Here you will find ball massage techniques and pelvic floor stretches to ease cramping and help you isolate pelvic floor contractions.

After a few rounds of happy baby and puppy dog stretching, lie on your back with your knees bent. Allow your legs to open like a butterfly and hold them here or rest them on cushions at either side.

From here exercise your pelvic floor in synchronisation with your breathing; breathe out as you close and lift your pelvic floor, breathe in as you release. Nice, long and slow breaths in and out up to ten times.

Next try some holds. Know that your endurance may not be great this week so stop when your muscles start to feel tired. Breathe out as you close and lift your pelvic floor, then take shallow breaths in and out as you hold up to ten seconds, before releasing on a slow breath in.

Finish with a few more stretches from task 3, your pelvic floor and menstruating body will thank you!

Week 2 – follicular phase: Getting ready for egg release comes with a rise in our sex hormone levels and a boost in energy. Stamina may still be fairly low, but take advantage of this fresher feeling to get stuck into your pelvic floor exercises. Find time each day to complete a full set of exercises to fatigue, including both endurance holds and faster isolated contractions. I recommend:

- Isolate your back passage, vaginal canal and urethra in turn. Work on all three layers of muscle at each canal, starting at the outside, then the middle and then the deepest layer. Alternate between the passages and hold for 10-20 seconds and up to ten of each.

- Now work on the same muscular contraction, but faster. Close and lift all three layers in one second and then release in one second. Repeat as quickly as you can, but be sure you relax fully in between each repetition. Aim for 10 fast lifts for the back, middle and front passages. If you need a re-cap on technique visit task 4 on page 58.

Week 3 – ovulatory phase: Your body has been building up to this phase, and your oestrogen and energy reach a simultaneous peak. Now is the time to work at your highest intensity and capitalise on this.

Functional pelvic floor exercises are a great way to make the most of this time. Incorporate your best pelvic floor contraction into exercises you enjoy. Combine your pelvic floor exercises into circuits at home – include some pelvic floor squats, press-ups and calf raises. As you press up from the floor, exhale, close and lift the pelvic floor at the same time. Release the contraction as you return to the start. You can use this principle in other exercises too: lunges, band work and weight lifting will all feel much stronger when you add the pelvic floor energy.

You can find and follow several series of exercises combined with pelvic floor contractions in task 5: Kettle bell kegels on page 67.

Week 4 – luteal phase: Coming out of your energy high may hit you suddenly or gradually over a few days. Your body is reaching the end of a cycle and already getting ready for the next one. Progesterone reaches its peak, so it's a good time to consolidate your strength training.

Take the movement of squats and exercise away and instead add some static resistance to your pelvic floor to fire up as many muscles as you can without overloading them. Squeezing a ball between your knees and simultaneously working through a set of your best 10-second pelvic floor holds will feel good all over. Similarly, resistance bands around your legs while performing pelvic floor exercises in sitting is a great way to work the pelvic floor and buttock muscles at the same time or practise task 9; Raising the Floor, on page 118 for an 'uplifting' pelvic floor workout.

Understanding why things are happening makes it a lot easier to fix them, so it's a good idea to get to know your cycle. You can anticipate your trickier days if you know what's around the corner. There are heaps of apps you can use or just put pen to paper to record your symptoms and plot your hormonal highs and lows.

When to ask for help:

- Experiencing unusually heavy or painful periods that you struggle to control with normal pad and tampon/cup usage.
- If you notice bleeding between your periods.

What to ask for:

- Hormonal tracking blood tests to detect levels which are too high, too low or not changing when they should.
- A referral to a gynaecologist to discuss and better understand hormonal control.

What's important

- Sex hormone inbalance post-partum is normal and can stay altered for six weeks or more after stopping breast feeding.
- Get some strength in the bank to avoid the impact of monthly fluctuating hormones on your pelvic floor.
- Once you have healed and rebuilt your strength after pregnancy and birth, mix up your pelvic floor exercises throughout the month to suit the challenges of each phase.

14. Preparing to go again: Strength enough for your hopes and dreams

Future pregnancies, or rather future births and recoveries, are either the first or last thing women ask me about. I often hear 'When will I be strong enough to cope with another pregnancy?', 'Should I have a Caesarean next time?' or 'Will this get worse if I have another baby?' When it's the first thing women ask me I know immediately that they feel broken. That something they had never considered possible happened to their bodies, and now their future hopes and dreams for their family have changed. When it is the last thing they ask me, after many months of healing, rebuilding and working together to recover, I know that they are beginning to feel fixed. What seemed impossible is suddenly within reach once more and feels achievable.

When these same women return to tell me they are pregnant again and ask for support along this next journey it is often with a mixture of excitement and fear. I tell them the hardest thing is done: the leap of faith in knowing you and your body can do this to embrace the idea of becoming pregnant again. Now you are here, and how much stronger are you going into this pregnancy knowing all that you know now? Prevention is always better than cure and we are going to do all we can to prepare for your recovery after this baby's birth before they've even arrived. We start now.

After the long road recovering from birth injuries, pelvic organ prolapse or pregnancy-related incontinence it is understandable to be fearful of undertaking this journey again. But let me tell you that the evidence concludes that you are not guaranteed another difficult birth nor birth injury just because it happened before. If we take pelvic organ prolapse as an example, there is only a 6% increase of prolapse with a second vaginal birth and almost no increase in reported symptoms.

Similarly, bladder weakness, bowel incontinence and pelvic floor trauma are not a given with subsequent births. Assisted deliveries, as in those with forceps or ventouse, carry greater risk of these injuries over the risk of further pregnancies and births alone.

In normal standing there is a pressure on our pelvic floor of around 37N. In the pushing stage of labour this can increase to 120N with each contraction. But this is still not as much force as when we cough or sneeze. While labour lasts longer than the average cough or sneeze, these strong explosive actions exert up to 129N on our pelvic floors and, as you have learnt, we can train them to withstand this. Often with first vaginal deliveries assistance of ventouse or forceps is required. The suction effect of ventouse comes with just 113N of force compared to 200N with forceps. This is a big jump up from the forces we have trained our pelvic floors to cope with and it's no wonder that this can lead to pelvic floor trauma and dysfunction. However these surgical procedures are performed in the best interests of mother and baby and there is sadly no way of knowing who will require this invasive assistance to birth 'naturally'. It is worth knowing, though, that if you had a ventouse or forceps delivery with your first birth there is an 80% chance you will deliver your next baby naturally, without the need for these procedures.

Pelvic and in particular pubic pain, however, is reported more frequently and earlier in subsequent pregnancies than the first. This does not mean the injury is bigger, but you are likely to notice pain and discomfort earlier in subsequent pregnancies if you experienced this with your first baby. So we need to consider our protect, stabilise and rehabilitate approach more than ever here and employ all you have learned about pelvic symmetry and the best exercises to keep your pelvis strong and stable for as long as possible.

Physiotherapy input will be valuable through this and subsequent pregnancies. Ask your GP for an early referral based on your symptoms in previous pregnancies so that you have access to help and physical therapy when you need it.

Vaginal birth after Caesarean (VBAC)

Whereas one vaginal birth significantly increases our risk of prolapse, Caesarean births are not associated with this same injury. Those who have

Caesarean births are less likely to experience a pelvic organ prolapse. Bladder and bowel incontinence is also more of a risk with vaginal birth than it is with abdominal births. While a Caesarean does not protect us from these injuries it does make them less likely. These are significant considerations when contemplating a vaginal birth after a Caesarean (VBAC) and you should discuss this with your midwife and obstetrician to better understand the risks of subsequent Caesareans compared to vaginal delivery after Caesarean section.

As I've said, for some reason society leads us to believe that vaginal birth comes with some sort of medal, but it really doesn't – unless we count prolapse as one! You do not need to give birth via your vagina to qualify as a mother, nor does opting for a Caesarean qualify as 'the easy route'. Caesarean comes with its own significant risks and it is important to fully understand those of a vaginal birth and an abdominal birth so that you can make an informed decision.

When weighing up the risks of a planned Caesarean section compared with a planned vaginal birth there is much to consider. You might find this list taken from the National Institute for Clinical Excellence (NICE) guidelines helpful, informative and maybe more than a little shocking:

Planned Caesarean section may reduce the risk of the following in women:

- Pain in the area between your vagina and anus (perineum) and in your abdomen (tummy) during birth and three days afterwards.
- Injury to your vagina.
- Heavy bleeding after birth.
- Anaemia and shock caused by loss of blood.

Planned Caesarean section may increase the risk of the following in women:

- Longer hospital stay.
- Bleeding after the birth that needs a hysterectomy (removal of the womb).
- Heart attack.

If you choose to have a VBAC you will be cared for in a maternity unit where a Caesarean section can be done very quickly if needed and where there are blood transfusion services. This is because there is a risk of uterine rupture (a tear of your womb) during labour after a previous abdominal birth. While this is very rare, you will be monitored carefully and cared for to check for this.

When you and your doctor are discussing whether to plan a Caesarean section or a vaginal birth, your doctor should take account of your preferences and priorities, the risks and benefits of another Caesarean section, and the risks and benefits of a VBAC. It's important that you feel listened to, considered and involved in this decision-making.

Many ideals exist around 'natural birth' with much focus given to mental preparation, which is important, but in my opinion there is not enough attention given to our physical preparation or, more specifically, the prevention of birth injuries. With nine out of ten first-time births resulting in some sort of medical intervention it's time we think of this as the norm and not the dreamy, relaxed, Mother Nature birth we are taught to expect. In my mind preparation and education is empowering. How often do we hear, 'My birth didn't go to plan'? But what if we change the plan? The plan is to prepare for, reduce the risk of and prevent if we can perineal tears or needing an episiotomy or medical assistance to birth. We know that there is a 90% chance that one or all of these may happen. What if we do all we can to be in that 10%? And if we all do this, who knows, maybe together with this knowledge and power we can even reverse these statistics. Here's how:

Perineal massage preparation: From 37 weeks this is a great way to prepare our bodies and minds for the stretch and pain that is to come when our baby's head is crowning. If you've been there then you know the perineal and vaginal discomfort I'm referring to. I will always remember my sister calling it 'the ring of fire'.

Perineal massage can prepare your body for this in two ways: by moisturising, stretching and promoting elasticity so that the skin of your perineum and vaginal opening can stretch more easily. By familiarising yourself with the soreness of your vaginal opening stretching, so that when this comes in birth you are prepared for it and can breathe and allow your body to stretch slowly. If it is a surprise, we tend to be fearful. If the pain is overwhelming we may rush this phase and push our baby out too quickly, which can increase our chances of tearing. Therefore perineal massage is considered an important step in birth preparation. Task 6 on page 83 will take you through the method for this. You can also try vaginal dilators or an Epi-No (as in 'no episiotomy'!), which is an inflatable device you can use to stretch your birth canal and vaginal opening with the same effects.

Positioning: Gravity is great for helping your baby descend and may reduce the time you spend pushing, which can in turn result in less trauma to your pelvic floor. If it is possible, try to be on your feet through your labour as much as you can and even opt for a squat position to birth in which naturally stretches your vaginal opening. If you are induced or you have an epidural in place then this may not be possible and you will need to labour and birth from bed. If this is the case, ask for a side lying position with your top leg supported open to mimic the same position as a squat.

Warm compress: Heat is another way to encourage your tissues to stretch and so is particularly valuable in birth. A warm bath or birthing pool is a great way to help all the muscles and ligaments of your pelvis and pelvic floor stretch slowly. Again, this may not always be possible and in this case warm compresses are recommended. Your midwife or birth partner can help you with this by applying a warm towel intermittently (it's really important it's not too hot) directly to your perineum during your second stage of labour.

Splinting: There are many surprising ways I can link the body to opening a bottle of wine and this is one of them! You can splint your perineum to make your baby's exit through your vagina much smoother and 'cleaner'. Much like holding down a bottle of wine as you ease the cork out. The firmer you hold it down and provide counter pressure, then the easier it is to draw the cork out. If you don't push back against the bottle firmly enough then it may lift and come with you as you draw back the cork.

Now make an L shape with your left hand and imagine placing this up against another person's perineum with the corner made of the webbing of your thumb around their vaginal opening. With a firm pressure here their perineum has a second layer of support from your hand to keep it still and intact as the baby presses down from the inside. Now imagine your midwife or birth partner's hand doing this job for you. This is a recommended birthing strategy to reduce the chances of perineal tearing and has already been adopted by many midwifes, but you may want to check that yours is happy to do this for you or get comfortable with the idea of doing this yourself.

Approaching this birth differently

Whichever birth you or your baby chooses, the most important part of your health and healing is the before and after. Approaching subsequent pregnancies with strength is important for a smooth recovery after birth. Consider your strength between your pregnancies as your new baseline rather than how you felt before your babies. If you restore your strength, regardless of your injuries, then you can confidently approach subsequent pregnancies and births knowing you can get back to here again. Knowledge is your strength. Knowing exactly what and how to heal and rebuild is your key to moving, feeling and living stronger after this and as many more babies as you choose to have.

Use these flow charts to tick off all you need to prepare and feel stronger. Each will direct you to your essential tasks to heal and rebuild and those which you can progress to when ready.

TASK 21 FLOW CHARTS FOR MOVING, FEELING AND LIVING STRONGER AFTER PREGNANCY AND BIRTH

Navigate the why and get straight to the rehabilitation with these flow diagrams summarising your rebuilding plan. Select the pathway that most suits your symptoms, bearing in mind that you may need to incorporate more than one flowchart. Combine those that cover your bothersome issues to create your own unique flow chart of where to start, what to progress on to and how to maintain your new found strength. This is where you can fast track to 'how to fix this'.

KIT YOU WILL NEED: This book!

Just to recap our tasks:

1. Finding the floor of your pelvis: page 30
2. Standing taller, living stronger: page 39
3. Let it go: page 55
4. Pelvic floor exercises for life: page 58
5. Kettle bell Kegels: page 67
6. Perineal massage, how-to guide: page 83

WHAT BOTHERS YOU THE MOST?

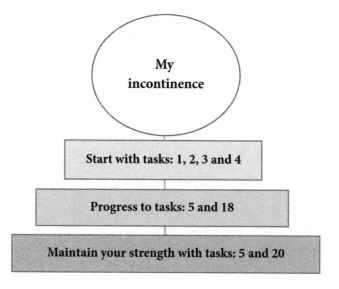

My incontinence

Start with tasks: 1, 2, 3 and 4

Progress to tasks: 5 and 18

Maintain your strength with tasks: 5 and 20

WHAT BOTHERS YOU THE MOST?

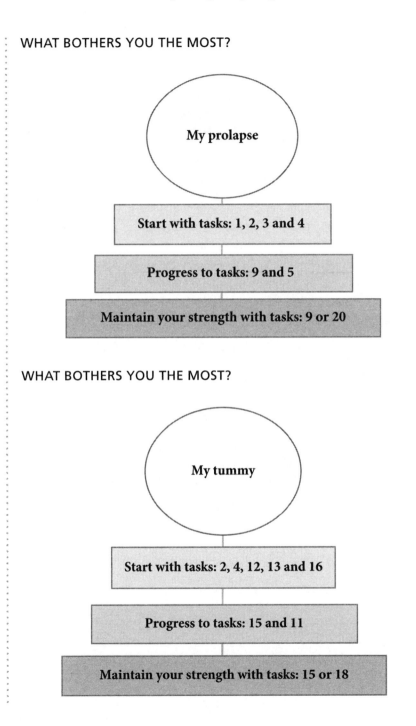

My prolapse

Start with tasks: 1, 2, 3 and 4

Progress to tasks: 9 and 5

Maintain your strength with tasks: 9 or 20

WHAT BOTHERS YOU THE MOST?

My tummy

Start with tasks: 2, 4, 12, 13 and 16

Progress to tasks: 15 and 11

Maintain your strength with tasks: 15 or 18

WHAT BOTHERS YOU THE MOST?

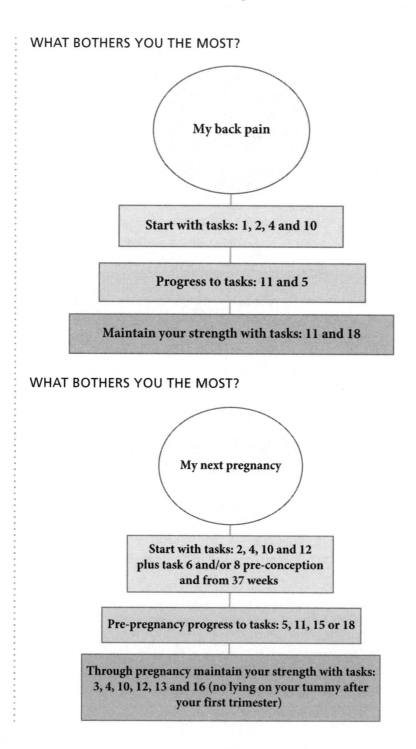

My back pain

Start with tasks: 1, 2, 4 and 10

Progress to tasks: 11 and 5

Maintain your strength with tasks: 11 and 18

WHAT BOTHERS YOU THE MOST?

My next pregnancy

Start with tasks: 2, 4, 10 and 12
plus task 6 and/or 8 pre-conception
and from 37 weeks

Pre-pregnancy progress to tasks: 5, 11, 15 or 18

Through pregnancy maintain your strength with tasks:
3, 4, 10, 12, 13 and 16 (no lying on your tummy after
your first trimester)

My story – baby number two

After the injuries I sustained in my first birth I was scared to face that trauma again. While I longed for more children the idea of birth filled me with dread. We both knew our daughter would love a sibling, but pregnancy and childbirth was too daunting a challenge. It took three years to rebuild strength in both my body and mind to tackle this again and still, throughout the pregnancy, the anxiety surrounding birth didn't leave me. I spoke openly about this at my ante-natal appointments. My midwife listened when I said, 'I can't think about giving birth. I just want her to stay inside me forever. I want to close my eyes for a few days while that bit is done and wake up after the event with her safely in my arms.' She referred me to a consultant midwife. I was nervous that day and prepared by scouring midwifery journals for the latest research. The time I had given my body to process and recover from my first birth empowered me to do all I could to avoid trauma the second time around.

Having this appointment was the best thing I could have done. We discussed the safest birth positions and agreed I would not be on my back this time, but on all fours or squatting to help my baby descend without medical intervention. If I needed help to birth her this would be tried first lying on my side to protect my perineum. We talked about splinting my perineum and how to do this (something I had learnt from the journals – if we or our midwife supports our perineum when our baby is crowning then we are less likely to tear). Lastly, we covered pushing – my biggest fear. After spending so long lifting everything back up and in, I couldn't imagine pushing my baby out. I didn't even think my body would remember how. The consultant midwife listened and reassured me. She had read the same research as me and agreed that excessive pushing and pushing too early could increase my risk of prolapse and stress incontinence. Instead, I should follow only my body's reactions. My body would expel my baby with its own pushing forces all on its own. I didn't need to push, bear down or strain, my body would know what to do. And it did.

Second time around my labour came in full force rather than bit by bit like my first. After seven hours of contractions, vomiting and pain I was dilated enough for the birthing pool. I was able to squat in the pool, supported by the water, to stretch my pelvic outlet and help her drop down, and the warmth of the water aided this too. But still, this bit was slow. I was letting my body do what it needed to, but I could still feel some resistance. I was holding on and consequently holding my baby in.

Finally, it had taken too long and I needed to get out of the water. With one leg in and one leg out, halfway to the bed, I was determined I could do this differently to last time. I didn't want to be on the bed with cuts and interventions. I was told to push hard and bear down in the end as my baby's heart rate was becoming erratic, but I tried to stay calm and understand why. So on my next contraction, half way out of the pool, I pressed up against my own perineum to give my baby something firmer to push against and emerge. With my hands here I could feel what was happening. She was stuck, the top of her head was out, but her chin was caught and perilously stretching my perineum, so I used my hand to scoop under her chin and free it before I tore. The rest of her body followed quickly then and I had no tears.

I kind of got my natural water birth – one leg was in the water at least! I am grateful that I entered my second birth more aware of what my body needed to do and how to protect myself. This story empowered me to share all I have learnt with you. Knowledge is power and should be available to every one of us.

When to ask for help:

- You need more support or advice in order to make informed choices about your birth.
- You are fearful or anxious about birth. You need to address this before the day comes.

What to ask for:

- An appointment with a consultant midwife or obstetric doctor. These are offered routinely when the mother has undergone a Caesarean first time around in order to prepare her for VBAC, but I strongly feel every mother should get a chance to discuss her options following a previous birth. Understanding all that happened in our first labour can unlock what we need to birth more easily next time around. We know now what labour and birth feels like; we have greater power and control to birth safely.

What's important

- Every birth is unique. Trauma in our first does not mean to say that this is inevitable in our second.
- You should feel supported to make informed choices about your birth first time, this time and every time.
- No one method of birth is superior to another.
- Birthing in a squatting position, on all fours and side-lying can reduce your chances of tearing.
- Avoid strenuous pushing and bearing down to protect yourself from urinary incontinence and prolapse down the line.
- Prepare for birth with perineal massage, just as in task 6, and especially if you have had a tear or episiotomy previously.
- Have faith in your body and its strength. You can do this.

15. Goals: Move, feel, live stronger

Stronger (adjective):
1 *Having the power to perform physically demanding tasks.*
2 *Able to withstand force, pressure, or wear.*
3 *Difficult to break, destroy or make sick.*

Strength is about feeling more capable, having a body that is resilient and tackles challenges with ease, and it goes far beyond the physical. The strength of our body and mind can be both what motivates us and what rewards us. Achieving and maintaining strength are not just training objectives, but goals for ourselves and our families, and for mothers especially.

We've seen the rise of the This Girl Can movement in sport, but the truth is many of us struggle to feel strong enough for everyday challenges. For many mothers feeling strong means being able to lift our baby, wear them in a sling or run after our toddler. Feeling stronger may be being able to return to work or to sport after growing and birthing a baby, or just having a pelvic floor which defies the 'bladder weakness' adverts. Strength can mean having the resilience to tackle the legacy of pregnancy and birth following the trauma of baby loss.

My main aim in bringing this book to you is to make strength after pregnancy and birth accessible to every mother and not just those who find themselves in the right hands. But if just getting through this book is daunting and seems a challenge too far, know that you don't have to do it all. What if you make just one change and you feel just 10% better? Every little change can be an improvement. You can pick this up and put it down as life dictates. Don't let too little time stop you from starting, even if it stops you continuing, and come back any time you need me.

It doesn't matter when you start this journey. It doesn't need to be straightaway to be most successful. If we haven't tried, we will never know. Not progressively loaded your pelvic floor since you had your children 10 years ago? Let's do it now. Didn't rehab your diastasis recti abdominis muscle after your first? Let's start now you're pregnant with your second. We can do this *now*. You don't need to wait until you've finished your family to begin. Just as each person's rehab is unique, every post-partum recovery is too. Your body may need something different after your second baby than it did after your first. Heal and rebuild as much as you can between your babies so that you enter each new phase as strong as you can.

Afterall, when does the rehab journey really end? Aren't we forever post-partum? Who knows what we could achieve if we keep going?

I do encourage you to seek the support of women's health physiotherapists, massage therapists, nutritionists, exercise specialists, gynaecologists, urogynaecologists, doctors and friends, whenever you can and whenever you need. They are all there to support you and your unique journey.

The words 'move', 'feel' and 'live stronger' adorn the walls of our rehabilitation space, Four Sides London, bringing the message that strength is achievable to all and that you can be strong enough, in both body and mind, throughout life and all its challenges. We are all so different and no two journeys will ever be the same, but there is so much overlap and I wanted to write this book to share all the advice I regularly pass onto my clients. I hope you find reasons, answers and solutions to better understand your post-natal body and that this gives you the keys to open the doors to your rehab and recovery.

References

Introduction

- 'Pelvic floor strengthening is low risk and the most effective way of resolving these issues '. 'Women's Health Physiotherapy is the number one treatment.' NICE 2019.

- '50% of pregnant women will experience lower back pain in pregnancy and, without treatment, 25% of those will still have pain one year after delivery.' Davenport et.al. 2019. Exercise for the prevention and treatment of low back, pelvic girdle and lumbopelvic pain during pregnancy: a systematic review and meta-analysis. *British Journal of Sports Medicine.* Volume 53, issue 2.

- '100% of women at full-term pregnancy will have some degree of tummy muscle overstretch and 30% will have a separation known as diastasis recti abdominis muscle'. Mota et.al. 2014. Prevalence and risk factors of diastasis recti abdominis from late pregnancy to 6 months postpartum, and relationship with lumbo-pelvic pain. *Manual Therapy.* 2014.09.002.

- '90% of first-time vaginal births will result in some degree of vagina or perineal tear and sometimes an episiotomy (a cut through the pelvic floor muscles to help the birth).' Dr Richmond. 2014. Perineal tearing is a national issue we must address. RCOG Blog. July 2014. www.rcog.org.uk/en/blog/perineal-tearing-is-a-national-issue-we-must-address.

- '25% of UK births are abdominal (via Caesarean section), which is major surgery.' Vogel et.al. 2015. Use of the Robson classification to assess Caesarean section trends in 21 countries: a secondary analysis of two WHO multi-country surveys. *Lancet Global Health.* 3:e260-e270.

- '3-7% of post-natal women will not be in full control of their bowels and will leak poo, while 25% will have no control over their wind (farting).' Eason et.al. 2002. Anal Incontinence after childbirth. *CMAJ* 2002;166(3):326-30. www.ics.org/publications/ici_5/incontinence.pdf.

- '30-50% of mums will wet themselves a little – or a lot'. Aoki et.al. 2017. *National Review Disease Primers*. 2017 Jul 6;3:17042.

- '50% of mothers will have some degree of pelvic organ prolapse by the time they reach menopause.' Gyhagen et al. 2012. Prevalence and risk factors for pelvic organ prolapse 20 years after childbirth: a national cohort study in singleton primiparae after vaginal or Caesarean delivery. *British journal of Obstetrics and Gynaecology*. 2012.

- 'Our emotional wellbeing has a big impact on how our bodies feel': Mazi et.al. 2019. Depression symptoms in women with pelvic floor dysfunction: a case-control study. *International Journal of Womens Health*. (11) pp.143–148.

- 'While more than a third of women suffer with urinary incontinence, only half of these will seek advice and treatment from medical professionals.' Melville et.al. 2008. Women's Perceptions about the Etiology of Urinary Incontinence. *J Womens Health (Larchmt)*. 2008 Sep; 17(7): 1093–1098.

1. Our bodies: My favourite parts

- 'The gap at the pubic symphysis is normally 3-4mm, but can more than double in pregnancy and birth to up to 9mm'. Rustamova et.al. 2009 Changes in Symphysis Pubis Width During Labor, *J Perinat Med*. 2009; 37(4):370-3.

- 'During pregnancy the ribcage can be stretched outwards by 4cm or more.' 'The ribcage is an anchor for the abdominal muscles and so the greater the increase in ribcage circumference during pregnancy, the wider and more significant the tummy muscle separation is.' Dr Sarah Duvall www. coreexercisesolutions.com/how-to-heal-a-diastasis-recti-without-surgery/.

- 'This is most common in multiple pregnancies or after several pregnancies and with increasing age, and is called a diastasis recti abdominis muscle (DRAM).' Thabet et al. 2019. Efficacy of deep core stability exercise programme in postpartum women with diastasis recti abdominis: a randomised controlled trial. *Journal of musculoskeletal neuronal interact*. 19(1): 62–68.

- 'Diane Lee, a physiotherapist and a role model of mine, has a similar analogy for our pelvic floor. She describes the pelvis as our door frame and the muscular pelvic floor as our door.' *A Clinical Guide for Those who are Split Down the Middle*. 2017. Published by Learn with Dianne Lee.

2. Posture: Strike a pose

- 'these four curves make our spines the strong and capable scaffolding that we rely on, allowing us to bend and flex. If we change the shape, position or depth of these curves, then we change the co-ordination, timing and strength of our muscular walls and we might find it harder to bend, flex or absorb everyday loads. This can make the movement we take for granted in our daily lives more effortful and even painful.' Dianne Lee. 2006. Pelvic stability and your core.pdf. www.scribd.com/document/423205624/2PelvicStability-Yourcore-pdf

3. The pelvic floor: You didn't know how good it was until it wasn't

- 'It's not surprising that post-pregnancy pelvic floor problems are closely linked to feelings of low self-esteem, poor quality of life and even post-natal depression.' Swenson *et.al.* 2018. Postpartum depression screening and pelvic floor symptoms among women referred to a specialty postpartum perineal clinic. *Am J Obstet Gynecol.* 2018;218(3).

- 'We assess all muscles on their strength according to the Oxford scale. This was modified for the pelvic floor by a brilliant physio called Jo Laycock.' Jeanette Haslam and Jo Laycock. 2008. *Therapeutic Management of Incontinence and Pelvic Pain, Pelvic Organ Disorders.* Second edition. Springer.

- 'A disconnect between the nerve and muscle so that the contraction cannot get through. This can happen in the long second stage of delivery when the baby's head presses on the pelvic floor nerves inside the birth canal, numbing their sensation or action, or when there has been a manual intervention in the delivery, such as ventouse or forceps, following trauma, abuse or surgery.' Wallace et.al. (2019). Pelvic floor physical therapy in the treatment of pelvic floor dysfunction in women. *Current Opinion Obstetrics and Gynecology.* 31:000 – 000.

- 'An overstretch of the muscles and tendons beyond what they can tolerate. Like stretching an elastic band, the pelvic floor muscles can accommodate a stretch of up to three times their length. Beyond this, overstretch occurs and, just as with an elastic band, they will struggle to return to their previous length.' Ashton-Miller, James A, and John O L Delancey. 2009.

On the biomechanics of vaginal birth and common sequelae. *Annual Review of Biomedical Engineering.* Vol. 11: 163-76.

- 'Most pelvic floor symptoms arise when the pelvic floor is too lax or too tense. We need to be on the lookout for an imbalance of some kind'. Wallace et.al. (2019). Pelvic floor physical therapy in the treatment of pelvic floor dysfunction in women. *Current Opinion Obstetrics and Gynecology.* 31:000 – 000.

- 'Post-traumatic stress disorder (PTSD) following a difficult birth is a very real thing and is diagnosed in 9% of us following childbirth.' Beck CT, Gable RK, Sakala C, Declercq ER. 2011. Posttraumatic stress disorder in new mothers: results from a two-stage U.S. national survey. *Birth.* 38(3):216-227.

- 'When you suspect your pelvic floor is too tense it can be beneficial to engage in whole-body movement and relaxation (I give you a head start on this in task 3 on page 55). Yoga is a great way to stretch through the pelvic floor and let it go, connecting your body and mind to release and relaxation.' Jeanette Haslam and Jo Laycock. 2008. *Therapeutic Management of Incontinence and Pelvic Pain, Pelvic Organ Disorders.* Second edition. Springer.

- 'NMES is recommended when pelvic floor strength is grade 2 or below on the scale, so when there is an inconsistent pelvic floor muscle contraction, just a flicker or no palpable contraction.' NICE 2006 and 2019. www.nice. org.uk/guidance/ng123/chapter/Recommendations#physical-therapies.

4. Birth injuries: Those that you can't put a plaster on

- 'With nine out of 10 vaginal births in first-time mothers resulting in cuts or tears to the nether regions, it is not just newborn babies who need tender loving care following their arrival.' RCOG 2020, www.rcog.org.uk/ en/patients/tears/tears-childbirth/.

- 'While an episiotomy isn't guaranteed to protect you from a perineal tear, it does make one less likely.' NHS. March 2020. www.nhs.uk/comditions/ pregnancy-baby/episiotomy.

- 'Perineal tears are graded according to their depth and what structures are involved...' RCOG 2020, www.rcog.org.uk/en/patients/tears/tears-childbirth/

- 'Take sitz baths'. www.whattoexpect.com/first-year/postpartum-health-and-care/sitz-bath-postpartum/

5. Abdominal birth recovery: Healing what we cannot see

- 'As 75% of Caesarean births are unplanned, many of you reading this won't have thought much about how a Caesarean goes before you suddenly found yourself having one.' www.ncbi.nlm.nih.gov/pmc/articles/PMC4907743/.

- 'Following a Caesarean section DRAM is most likely to be found below your tummy button, directly where your muscles were stretched, whereas following a vaginal birth DRAM is more likely to be found at and above your navel.' www.ncbi.nlm.nih.gov/books/NBK546707/.

- 'Silicone strips are recommended to reduce excessive scarring and minimise scar appearance.' www.nhs.uk/conditions/scars/treatment/.

6. Prolapse: The silent epidemic

- 'Mothers who are induced are more likely to need some help, such as ventouse or even forceps, delivering the baby's head.' www.nhs.uk/conditions/pregnancy-and-baby/induction-labour/.

- 'Approximately 5% of us have one or more hypermobile joints. Hypermobility syndrome is a diagnosis given to those of us who are super-bendy or double-jointed.' www.en.wikipedia.org/wiki/Hypermobility_syndrome.

- 'This sort of prolapse is most likely to occur after childbirth and up to a third of women who experience traumatic births, such as my first experience, will sustain an injury to their anterior vaginal wall.' Hans Peter Dietz. 2013. Pelvic Floor Trauma in Childbirth. *Australian and New Zealand Journal of Obstetrics and Gynaecology.* 53; 220-230.

- 'You may well have heard, and consequently become terrified of, vaginal surgery whereby mesh has been routinely used to support a prolapsed uterus. This 'engineering' has been getting a lot of bad press recently and rightly so. Although it has been successful in reducing prolapse symptoms and was the gold standard surgery for pelvic organ prolapse for years, it has been found that over time the mesh can work its way free and into a woman's bladder, bowel or vagina, causing considerable pain and discomfort ... this type of surgery is no longer recommended due to its 'serious but well-recognised safety concerns." www.nice.org.uk/guidance/ipg599/resources/transvaginal-mesh-repair-of-anterior-or-posterior-vaginal-wall-prolapse-pdf-1899872237521861.

- 'Oestrogen creams and pessaries can be prescribed by your doctor to help with the healing of prolapse while breastfeeding.' breastfeeding-and-medication.co.uk/fact-sheet/breastfeeding-and-oestrogen-cream-or-pessary.

7. Pelvic pain: Re-centring the keystone to strength

- 'Risk factors for SPD include...' www.ncbi.nlm.nih.gov/books/NBK537043/ and www.ncbi.nlm.nih.gov/pmc/articles/PMC5702981/#r3
- 'incontinence in late-stage pregnancy that can remain a problem years later'. Sangsawang B, Sangsawang N. 2013. Stress urinary incontinence in pregnant women: a review of prevalence, pathophysiology, and treatment. *International Urogynecology Journal.* 24(6):901-912.

8. Tummy recovery: We've fixed the floor, but what about the walls?

- 'When our tummy muscles are split down the middle we are much more likely to experience back pain, wet knickers and even pelvic organ prolapse. And it's not just physical symptoms that post-baby tummy changes gift us, but also damaging effects on our body confidence.' Wang, Q., Yu, X., Chen, G. et al. 2020. Does diastasis recti abdominis weaken pelvic floor function? A cross-sectional study. *Int Urogynecol J.* 31, pp.277–283. Parker M, Millar L, Dugan S. 2009. Diastasis rectus abdominis and lumbo-pelvic pain and dysfunction – Are they related? *Journal of Women's Health Physical Therapy.* 33(2): pp.15-22.
- 'This gap is necessary to provide space for our baby to grow but should close again within eight weeks of giving birth (abdominal or otherwise). One in three mums will notice that their gap takes longer to close than this, and this can be a result of diastasis recti abdominis muscle (DRAM), which literally translates as separated rectus abdominis muscle...' Coldron Y, Stokes M J, Newham D J et al. 2008. Postpartum characteristics of rectus abdominis on ultrasound imaging. *Manual Therapy.* 13: 112.

- 'One study asked physios about their experiences in supporting women who had been living with DRAM for more than two years and specifically if there was still the opportunity for improvement. Every physio agreed that there is some degree of recovery, whether you start retraining at six, 60 or 600+ weeks post-pregnancy and birth'. Keeler, Jessica et.al. 2012. Diastasis Recti Abdominis: A Survey of Women's Health Specialists for Current Physical Therapy Clinical Practice for Postpartum Women. *Journal of Women's Health Physical Therapy*. 36:3 pp. 131-142.

9. Breathing: Firing up your engine

- 'In weeks 2 to 5 we see our heart rate increase by 16 to 20 beats per minute, often before we even know we are expecting.' Gabbe Steven G: 2012. *Obstetrics: Normal and Problem Pregnancies*. Sixth edition. Saunders. chapter 3: Maternal Physiology, 42-65.

- 'As our body and growing baby continue to demand more oxygen we take in 30-40% more air with every breath we take.' LoMauro, Antonella, and Andrea Aliverti. 2015. 'Respiratory physiology of pregnancy: Physiology masterclass. *Breathe* (Sheffield, England) vol. 11,4: 297-301.

- 'Relaxin reaches its peak in trimester 2, which is when pelvic, back and rib pain are more likely.' Dehghan, F et al. 2014. The effect of relaxin on the musculoskeletal system. *Scandinavian journal of medicine & science in sports*. vol. 24,4: e220-9.

- 'As our baby seems to fill our entire abdomen our ability to take a full breath is down by 20% as we have less space to breathe deeply'. 'As our baby reaches full term our diaphragm is pushed upwards and our ribcage is forced outwards by 4cm or more.' LoMauro A, Aliverti A. 2015. Respiratory physiology of pregnancy: Physiology masterclass. *Breathe* (Sheffield). 11(4):297-301.

- '10-15kg of total weight gain is expected'. Institute of Medicine (US) Committee on Nutritional Status During Pregnancy and Lactation. 1990. Nutrition During Pregnancy: Part I Weight Gain: Part II Nutrient Supplements. Washington (DC): National Academies Press (US). Total Amount and Pattern of Weight Gain: Physiologic and Maternal Determinants. Available from: www.ncbi.nlm.nih.gov/books/NBK235227/

- 'In simple terms hypopressives require you to breathe out fully and hold for as long as you can before breathing in again. The truth is incorporating breath training alongside pelvic floor muscle re-training is what leads to the greatest success in reducing symptoms of incontinence and prolapse.' Pelvic Floor Muscle Training Is Better Than Hypopressive Exercises in Pelvic Organ Prolapse Treatment: An Assessor-Blinded Randomized Controlled Trial. 2019. *Neurourology Urodynamics.* 38(1):171-179.

10. Fuelling your journey: What goes in must come out

- USDA National Nutrient Database 2015.

11. Sports and exercise: For body and mind

- 'We are all recommended to be physically active every day and spend at least 150 minutes a week on moderate intensity exercise, even in pregnancy, before even becoming pregnant and forever more.' www.nhs.uk/live-well/exercise/

- B. K. Pedersen & B. Saltin. 2015. Exercise as medicine – Evidence for prescribing exercise as therapy in 26 different chronic diseases. *Scand J Med Sci Sports.* (Suppl. 3) 25: 1–72.

- 'The American College of Sports Medicine has outlined exactly what types of exercise are best and exactly what our routine should entail...' ACSM's Guidelines for Exercise Testing and Prescription. 2017. American College of Sports Medicine.

- 'I understand that this can feel daunting, and you are not alone. More than half of us aren't able manage to find the time and space to incorporate daily exercise and a quarter of us feel unable to exercise at all'. Senter et.al. 2013. Prescribing exercise for women. *Current Review of Musculoskeletal Medicine.* 6 (2) 164-172.

- 'The power of exercise to heal a worried mind has been hugely documented and is recommended for stress, anxiety, depression and more'. Tsatsoulis and Fountoulakis. 2006. The Protective Role of Exercise on Stress System Dysregulation and Comorbidities. *Annals of the New York Academy of Sciences.* Volume 1083, issue 1.

- 'The return to running after pregnancy and birth has been given much attention and thankfully we can now find exact return to run criteria in the research'. Groom, Donnelly and Brockwell. 2019. *Returning to Running Postnatal – guidelines for medical, health and fitness professionals managing this population.*

12. Intimacy: Pleasure, connection and sex

- '78% of women will not climax with penetrative sex alone and need clitoral stimulation to reach the big O. Shockingly one sex study has found that 100% of men climax from penis in vagina sex, compared to 10% of women'. Brody and Weiss. 2010. Vaginal Orgasm Is Associated With Vaginal (Not Clitoral) Sex Education, Focusing Mental Attention on Vaginal Sensations, Intercourse Duration, and a Preference for a Longer Penis. *Journal of Sexual Medicine.* (8):2774-81.

- 'Intimate touch, orgasms and early pelvic floor exercises will help to heal and rebuild your nerves and the muscles'. *Rieder B. 2016. Role of Pelvic Floor Muscles in Female Orgasmic Response. Journal of Women's Health Issues. Care 5:6.*

13. Hormones: The good, the bad and the monthly

- 'Some truths about "women's hormones"'. www.medlineplus.gov/hormones.html and www.en.wikipedia.org/wiki/List_of_human_hormones.

- 'the amazing phenomenon whereby women wear fewer clothes when they are ovulating as some sort of 'evolutionary call to procreate'. Kristina M. Durante, et.al. 2011. Ovulation, Female Competition, and Product Choice: Hormonal Influences on Consumer Behavior. *Journal of Consumer Research.* Volume 37, Issue 6, pp. 921–934.

- 'The pelvic floor, bladder and urethra contain oestrogen receptors, so we might not be aware of it, but oestrogen helps to maintain tone and tension in these muscles all the time'. Weber et.al. 2015. Local Oestrogen for Pelvic Floor Disorders: A Systematic Review. *PLos One.* 10 (9)s.

- 'Prolactin can have a knock-on effect on our happy hormone, dopamine. This gives us feelings of euphoria and happiness, which, as new mothers with our world in our arms, we probably have in abundance. But prolactin can hit dopamine levels hard and, together with less sleep than normal and a drop-off in oestrogen, these euphoric feelings can be hard to find and they can be replaced by low energy levels, sudden and extreme highs and lows, and even a slower metabolism for many months after birth.' www.medlineplus.gov/hormones.html and www.en.wikipedia.org/wiki/List_of_human_hormones

- 'It can take six to eight weeks after giving birth or stopping breastfeeding for our hormones to return to their normal balance'. Meaghan O'Connell. 2019. Life on Planet Weaning: I stopped breastfeeding and became a hormone detective. *The Cut: Science of us*. www.thecut.com/2019/07/what-happens-to-your-hormones-when-you-stop-breastfeeding.html.

14. Preparing to go again: Strength enough for your hopes and dreams

- 'there is only a 6% increase in evidence of prolapse with a second vaginal birth and almost no increase in reported symptoms.' Lieschen et.al. 2010. Vaginal Parity and Pelvic Organ Prolapse. *Journal of Reproductive Medicine*. 55(3-4): 93–98.

- 'In normal standing there is a pressure on our pelvic floor of around 37N. In the pushing stage of labour this can increase to 120N with each contraction. But this is still not as much force as when we cough or sneeze. While labour lasts longer than the average cough or sneeze, these strong explosive actions exert up to 129N on our pelvic floors and, as you have learnt, we can train them to withstand this. Often with first vaginal deliveries assistance of ventouse or forceps is required. The suction effect of ventouse comes with just 113N of force compared with 200N with forceps.'

  Ashton-Miller, James A, and John O L Delancey. 2009. On the biomechanics of vaginal birth and common sequelae. *Annual Review of Biomedical Engineering*. Vol. 11 (2009): 163-76.

- 'it is worth knowing ... that if you had a ventouse or forceps delivery with your first birth, there is an 80% chance you will deliver your next baby naturally, without the need for these procedures'. www.rcog.org.uk/globalassets/documents/patients/patient-information-leaflets/pregnancy/pi-an-assisted-vaginal-birth-ventouse-or-forceps.pdf.

References

- 'When weighing up the risks of a planned Caesarean section compared with a planned vaginal birth there is much to consider.' NICE clinical guideline [CG132] 2011 (updated 2019). www.nice.org.uk/guidance/cg132. Roberts & Hanson. 2007. Best Practices in Second Stage Labor Care: Maternal Bearing Down and Positioning. *J Midwifery Women's Health.* 52(3):238-45.

- 'Whereas one vaginal birth significantly increases our risk of prolapse, Caesarean births are not associated with this same injury. Those who have Caesarean birth are less likely to experience a pelvic organ prolapse. Bladder and bowel incontinence is also more of a risk with vaginal birth than it is with abdominal births. While a Caesarean does not protect us from these injuries it does make them less likely.' Lowdermilk et al. 2012. *Maternity and Women's Health Care,* 10th edition, chapter 19.

- 'A warm bath or birthing pool is a great way to help all the muscles and ligaments of your pelvis and pelvic floor stretch slowly. Again, this may not always be possible and in this case warm compresses are recommended.' www.royalberkshire.nhs.uk/patient-information-leaflets/Maternity/Preventing%20perineal%20tears_apr19.pdf.

Further reading and useful links

Find your own women's health physio:

- www.csp.org.uk/public-patient/find-physiotherapist/physio2u. In the first instance visit your GP and ask for what you need. While this can feel embarrassing, they want to help you and the more information you can give them, then the better this help will be. Insist on being heard, don't accept how you feel as 'normal' if it doesn't feel right for you. Women's health physiotherapy is nearly always the best place to start and if you want a more direct route than through your GP, visit the Chartered Society of Physiotherapy. Just pop in your postcode and find help nearby quickly.

Explore your body deeper

- www.postpartum.net. A wealth of information for mums and dads trying to understand what just happened in the labour room! Straightforward explanations of why, what and how.
- www.pelvichealthsolutions.ca/for-the-patient/what-is-pelvic-floor-physiotherapy/. A brilliant website I discovered when I lived and worked in Canada. I would often direct women here to work out what was driving their symptoms. It's particularly good for understanding more about high tone or a non-relaxing pelvic floor.
- *Period Power: Harness Your Hormones and Get Your Cycle Working for You* by Maisie Hill. For more on the magic of tracking our cycle and working with our body's natural rhythm.
- *More Orgasms Please: Why Female Pleasure Matters* by The Hotbed Collective. What's not to love about this! There can be no bigger challenge than pleasurable sex post-partum, but it is possible. You can get there and who doesn't want/need more orgasms please?!
- *Postnatal Pilates: A Recovery and Strength Guide for Life* by Anya Hayes. For more exercises to heal and rebuild after pregnancy and birth.

- *Diastasis Rectus Abdominis: A Clinical Guide for those who are Split Down the Middle* by Dianne Lee. If you are healing a DRAM you will want to read this or, if it is too heavy for you, you'll want your physio to!
- These two diagrams are quick visual guides to safely return to running after pregnancy and birth. Designed by physiotherapists Emma Brockwell, Grianne Donnelly and Tom Groom, these are super-helpful resources if running is your thing. www.blogs.bmj.com/bjsm/files/2019/05/IMG_4349. jpg www.blogs.bmj.com/bjsm/files/2019/05/IMG_4348.jpg

For solidarity, support and sharing:

- *PMSL: Or How I Literally Pissed Myself Laughing and Survived the Last Taboo to Tell the Tale* by Luce Brett. A funny, brilliant read about a serious business. Luce's account of her experiences with incontinence, physiotherapy and ultimately recovery after pregnancy and birth made me cry, smile, laugh and even change a thing or two about my physiotherapy. Like: where to direct women to put their knickers when undressing for a physical examination, especially if they're hoping to hide the 'just in case' pad inside. I now point out the chair for clothes and knickers or the basket for belongings if you prefer. Understanding we are not alone and observing others' experiences in recovery may be all we need to kickstart our own journeys in healing and rebuilding.
- Facebook. While an unlikely source, I have met many women who have found the support they needed here. Try searching groups for prolapse, incontinence and diastasis. You can even find local ones and build your own support group online or in person.

Getting ready to go again:

- *The Fourth Trimester: A Postpartum Guide to Healing Your Body, Balancing Your Emotions, and Restoring Your Vitality* by Kimberly Ann Johnson. A beautiful, friendly and informative read. Tips for you, your partner and your support network to prepare and heal both body and mind for pregnancy and birth.
- *Give birth like a feminist: Your Body, Your Baby, Your Choices* by Milli Hill. Practical advice on everything, including dealing with doctors and doulas,

so that you get what you need in pregnancy and birth. This call to arms is the only guide you need to stand and deliver, and get the birth that's right for you.

For head space:

- *Untamed: Stop Pleasing, Start Living* by Glennon Doyle. If you've not read this yet, please do. Start living.
- *The Boy, The Mole, The Fox and The Horse* by Charlie Mackesy. Such a lovely book to read together. Parts will resonate and feel like a hand to hold on this journey.

'Treat' yourself:

- Bottoms Up. A soothing, cooling and calming spray for your bits after birth. Naturalbirthingcompany.com.
- Spritz for Bits. Instant relief for perineal soreness and bruising. Myexpertmidwife.com They also do a great combo set which includes Peri Prep Your Bits for perineal massage in pregnancy and after birth.
- Perineal Mama Mist. Taken straight from their website: 'Yo Mama, well done. Birth is no joke. You've contained a universe, you've stretched big and looked your edge square in its eye. Time for some soothing and repair'. fatandthemoon.com.
- Vaginal Victory Oil and Scar Saviour for pre- and post-pregnancy skin hydration and nourishment. I love these products as much as their names! Nessaorganics.com.
- Prepare Elixir and Self Love Potion. Handcrafted, natural luxuries for birth preparation and sexual pleasure. Womanology.life.
- Neen Pelvic Floor Educator. This little indicator is a simple and cost-effective way to know if you're doing your pelvic floor exercises correctly. www.neenpelvichealth.com/products/Educator-r/.
- Core Shorts. For pelvis support when you return to exercise. www.coretection.com.

For more exercise that is safe, healing and rehabilitating you can follow my Pilates programmes at: www.foursideslondon.com/four-sides-at-home/. You will find a class for every month of future pregnancies to support your tummy and pelvic floor as well as prevention of back and pelvic pain. Also four short post-natal exercise videos, each with their own goal: Stretch and Release, Activation, Pelvic Ring Closure and Core Abdominals.

Acknowledgements

My thanks must start at the very beginning of this idea. It came about around a camp fire, sharing birth stories with my friend Dr Jane, a recently retired GP, she encouraged me to share all that I've learnt. Motivated by her words 'trust me women don't know this stuff and they deserve to', I started writing.

Over dinner at The Naughty Piglets our chef friend Joe introduced me to Bravo Blue agency and my ideas became a book under the guidance of Charlotte Colwill. With her help I became a writer as well as a physiotherapist.

Charlotte soon became known as 'My Charlotte', after meeting 'Bloomsbury Charlotte'. To both I owe a lot of thanks, their ideas, patience and encouragement brought the best out of me.

Thank you to my editor, Sarah, for all your advice. I loved and will miss our chats; thank you for listening. Together with Luisa (Stronger's beautiful cover artist) and Jasmine (talented illustrator) you brought my book to life.

To all of my friends patiently trawling through first drafts and your super helpful corrections and removals of exclamation marks; Lou, Ruth, James, Claire, Kasey, Carrie, Mum and Dad.

Behind all of this and me, every step of the way, my Robyn, Coco and James. Thank you. I was able to do this because of and thanks to you.

A big thank you to all of the women who entrusted me with their post-natal recoveries; your strength empowered me. If you're listening to the audio version of this book then you will hear the voice of Jo, whom I had the pleasure of supporting through two out of her three pregnancy and post-natal journeys. Thank you to Jo for being as excited to work on this project as I was to have you. Four Sides team, space and community has been the best platform I could have wished for and I am grateful for all that this has brought me and my family.

And lastly to Carrie. For keeping this authentically 'Meg' with your support, encouragement and love, thank you.

Index

Index

Index